Multiple Sclerosis

New Hope and Practical Advice for People with MS and Their Families

Revised and Updated Edition

Louis J. Rosner, M.D., and Shelley Ross

A FIRESIDE BOOK
Published by Simon & Schuster
New York London Toronto Sydney

Fireside
A Division of Simon & Schuster, Inc.
1230 Avenue of the Americas
New York, NY 10020

DISCLAIMER: As no two cases of multiple sclerosis present the same, progress the same, or respond to treatment in the same way, the reader should consult a board certified neurologist or other health care professional before acting on advice or information published in this book.

The author and publisher disclaim any liability arising directly or indirectly from the use of this book.

This Fireside trade paperback edition March 2008

FIRESIDE and colophon are registered trademarks of Simon & Schuster, Inc.

For information about special discounts for bulk purchases, please contact Simon & Schuster Special Sales at 1-800-456-6798 or business@simonandschuster.com.

Designed by Carla Jayne Little

Manufactured in the United States of America

10 9 8 7 6 5 4 3 2 1

Library of Congress Cataloging-in-Publication Data is available.

ISBN-13: 978-1-4165-5099-0
ISBN-10: 1-4165-5099-2

To Larraine R., who looks at science
with a human eye
And to all the patients who inspire
with their courage
—L. R.

To David S.
And to the researchers who toil in
laboratories around the world in search
of a cure for MS
—S. R.

Acknowledgments

Many people have helped, both directly and indirectly, with the publication of this book. First, we thank those who anonymously contributed to our realistic approach of the subject. Next, in deepest gratitude for inspiration and information, we thank Dr. Augustus Rose, professor emeritus of neurology at UCLA; Dr. Stephen Reingold, assistant vice-president for research and director of grants management for the National Multiple Sclerosis Society in New York; and Dr. Al Kerza-Kwiatecki, health scientist administrator for Demyelinating, Atrophic, and Dementing Disorders Program at the National Institute of Neurological and Communicable Disorders and Stroke (NINCDS). Also acknowledged are Thor Hanson, president and chief executive officer of the National Multiple Sclerosis Society, and the rest of his staff, including science editor Phyllis Shaw. Finally, we thank agent Barbara Lowenstein, editor Paul Aron, and friend Ellen Goodstein, who all greatly contributed to the timely publication of our book.

Contents

Preface

It's been twenty years since the first edition of this book came out—over fifty years that I've been personally involved with treatment of MS—and I finally have seen the revolution.

It was 1956, as a neurology resident in Houston, when I fell in love with a beautiful young ice-skater who had just been diagnosed with multiple sclerosis. In my naiveté, I vowed I would find a cure. Three years later, after a stint at the New York Neurological Institute, I moved to Los Angeles to take over the MS clinic at the UCLA Medical Center. Back then, the diagnosis of MS was very difficult to make and often took years. The cause was a mystery. And we could only dream of the day when new technology would offer some way to see the lesions in the brain and track the disease. Most frustrating of all, back then, there was no effective treatment to change the course of the disease.

Today, with MRI technology, the diagnosis can be made within days after onset. The cause is largely solved. And there is effective treatment available to everyone to change the course of the disease. All of this, in my lifetime.

Sadly, I learned the beautiful young ice-skater who had stayed behind in Houston, had died during experimental surgery for relief of severe tremor. If she came along now, she could be saved and probably would have no permanent damage. So while I honor the courage of those who battled MS in earlier times, I am grateful we have come so far so fast.

—Louis J. Rosner

I first met Dr. Louis Rosner in 1986, when his private medical office was right across the street from my apartment in Beverly Hills, where I had moved to pursue a writing and producing career in television. At the time, he told me he wanted to write a book for people with MS that would contain all the information he could provide if he moved in with his patients for two weeks to answer each and every question. I couldn't pass up such a unique—not to mention geographically convenient—project, so for the next six months we worked together in between his patients and my TV assignments. During our collaboration I got a very unique look at the challenges of living with a neurological deficit. Not just from Dr. Rosner's instruction or assignments to look up various journals at the UCLA biomedical library, but from his own example. Dr. Rosner—the neurologist with a quick wit, love of inventing crossword puzzles, and dedication to his beautiful wife, Larraine—has lived not with MS, but with the ravages of polio. He doesn't really ever talk about it, but as he clicks his leg braces in place to stand up, you know he knows. And you know when he gives guidance, it means something. You know when he is optimistic, it's real. And you know when he says "This is the revolution" in the treatment of MS, it is.

In the twenty years since the first edition of this book, I did become a television writer producer, winning three Emmy Awards, a Peabody Award, and more. I became executive producer at ABC's *Good Morning America* with Diane Sawyer and Charlie Gibson and executive producer of *Prime Time*

Live. I produced interviews with four U.S, presidents, one prime minister, and dozens of celebrities. I produced live two-hour specials from the White House after Columbine, from the Pentagon after September 11, from the Vatican on the occasion of the pope's twenty-fifth anniversary. Yet there isn't anything I've written or produced that has been as rewarding as this book. One of the most extraordinary experiences came after learning that my college roommate was diagnosed with MS. She described her neurologist as so pathologically uncomfortable in breaking the news, he couldn't say the words "multiple sclerosis." Instead she had to grab her file from his desk and read it herself. Our humble book, which would ultimately have her personal notes in almost every margin, would change her trauma into hope and action.

A few years after that, I got a phone call asking me to call a former colleague at *PrimeTime Live*: Lori Bores had been diagnosed with MS. I called the number and we chatted away for an hour. Little did I know I was calling Lori in the hospital. Her attack had been severe. But that didn't stop her from e-mailing me some time after: "Thank god I got the disease Shelley Ross wrote the book about." I spoke to Lori recently. She no longer works in network news, but she sounded as busy as ever and full of joy. She told me those early days informed the optimistic outlook she still has today. "Reading the case histories in your book, I knew: I can handle this." What a blessing to make a difference.

—Shelley Ross

1

MS—What Is It, Who Gets It, and Why

If ever a disease could be called fascinating, it would be multiple sclerosis. The volumes of available facts and figures give it an intriguing identity. We know, for example, that in the United States almost triple the number of MS cases are found above the thirty-seventh parallel (running from Santa Cruz, California, to Newport News, Virginia) as are found below it. In certain areas of the world, not a single case of MS has ever been reported. Certain races appear to be relatively immune. Some studies show that women from the upper echelons of society, aged twenty-five to thirty-five, form a noticeably high percentage of MS cases, a fact suggesting that MS is some kind of "elitist" disease. Why do all these facts consistently hold true? Scientists today are closing in on the answers to this and other perplexing questions.

We now know what MS is, who gets it, and when, where, and possibly why. Some aspects of the disease, however, such as its cause, still remain a mystery. In fact, a researcher once compared it to the old Indian legend in which a group of blind men encounter an elephant. They can each describe the part of the animal they have touched, but none of them can explain the total picture. This is the case with MS.

Still, scientists are closer than ever to describing the whole MS elephant. In January 1985 a team of researchers from Stanford University announced that they had wiped out a disease in mice that is similar to MS. We are truly on the threshold of discovery.

Among the general public, MS is one of the most misunderstood diseases. Just think of the public service slogan: MS, the Crippler of Young Adults. That's a pretty gloomy label for a disease where 75 percent of those who have it will never need a wheelchair. Whether you've just been diagnosed as having MS or you've lived with it a while—or even if the MS patient is someone you happen to care for—it's important to know that misinformation is a greater enemy than the disease itself. So, while we can't provide you with a cure in these pages, we can give you the best tools to beat MS—the facts.

The History

The MS story begins almost like a fairy tale, because once upon a time there was no MS—not a case was known to medicine. Then, in the 1830s, two doctors in Europe began to write of a "new" disease, one never seen before. Jean Cruveilhier, professor of pathological anatomy in the Faculty of Medicine at the University of Paris, is credited with the first clinical report in 1835. During routine autopsies, he observed some "brown patches" in the central nervous system and described them to the medical community. Simultaneously, Robert Carswell was commissioned by the museum at University College in London to show a collection of sketches of the central nervous system that he had drawn as a young medical student. Among the two thousand color pictures he had drawn while observing autopsies were some that included unexplained "spots." In 1838, Carswell published an atlas of his drawings, along with written descriptions. In one chapter he wrote, "The anterior surface of the spinal cord presented a number of spots, from a quarter of an inch to half an inch in breadth."

Both Cruveilhier and Carswell only observed the effects of the disease during autopsies. A German doctor named Friedrich Theodor von Frerichs is given credit for the first diagnosis of the disease in a living subject. In 1849 he published a report more similar to the modern concept of MS. He wrote that it is more common in younger patients, that it is characterized by slow progression, that one side of the body is affected and then the other, and so on.

At about this time, too, reports of this disease started to appear outside medical literature. Perhaps the most famous historical case is recorded in the diary and letters of Sir Augustus Frederick d'Este (1794–1848), a grandson of George III of England and a cousin of Queen Victoria. In his published papers, he described his twenty-five years with recurring symptoms that included blurred vision, loss of balance, numbness in the limbs, and paralysis.

Around the world isolated reports of this odd disease were cropping up, but it is the French neurologist Jean-Martin Charcot who is credited with bringing the first clear-cut description of multiple sclerosis to the attention of the medical world. Charcot, the foremost authority on paralysis in Europe, attracted doctors from all parts of the continent to his dramatic lectures and presentations. Among his prominent students was the young Sigmund Freud, who traveled from Vienna to observe Charcot's treatment of patients with "hysterical" paralysis—those paralyzed by emotional, not physical, problems. Charcot would actually get these patients to walk again by hypnotizing them, tricking them, or frightening them horribly. Freud, who became convinced that there were better ways to treat hysteria, ultimately went off on his own and pioneered psychoanalysis.

Still, what Charcot might have lacked in compassion he made up for in medical genius. In 1868 he identified a new disease that had previously been confused with paralysis. He was able to make his first observations of what would soon become known as multiple sclerosis right under his nose—his own housekeeper had the disease.

On March 14, 1868, Charcot presented the clinical aspects of three cases to the French Biological Society. Soon after, he presented his own illustrations of the disease—sketches that would appear in neurology textbooks for many generations to come. Most important, though, he was the first to correlate the "brown patches" discovered by Cruveilhier and Carswell with the symptoms of the disease he called *sclérose en plaques,* translated as "hardening in patches."

Because of Charcot's reputation and prominence, word of this new disease spread quickly, and the study of neurology would never be quite the same. Unfortunately, he only identified three symptoms of the disease—the ones he observed in his maid—and for years this led to very limited diagnosis around the world. In fact, until the 1950s the Japanese were thought to be immune to MS. They weren't immune at all; they had symptoms other than those in Charcot's literature, which was still respected as medical gospel.

The first American reports of MS began with a paper given on December 4, 1867, to the College of Physicians in Philadelphia, called "The Case of the Late Dr. C. W. Pennock." Dr. Pennock had been a physician trained both at the University of Pennsylvania and in Paris. Over a period of twenty-four years, he suffered progressive weakness and numbness in his limbs that left him unable to walk and ultimately to work. Dr. Pennock also noticed that warm weather made him feel weaker. His autopsy report mentioned "spots" that were discovered in the spinal cord. Although no name for the disease was ever given, it is apparent today that the case described was one of multiple sclerosis. It wasn't until 1878 that the term *sclerosis* appeared in American medical literature.

Our knowledge of MS is fairly new. As we look back now, the question is, Did MS appear out of the blue in the 1830s, or was it an older disease overlooked by doctors who made less acute observations? If it is a relatively new disease, it wouldn't be the first time in medical history a disease has suddenly appeared. Syphilis, for example, was unheard of before 1492, one of the more important dates we learn in elementary school. This is not a coincidence, since it was actually Christopher Columbus and his sailors who brought the disease to Europe. Syphilis was a very mild disease that was common among the women of Haiti. After Columbus's first voyage, he and his sailors returned to Europe via Haiti, where they contracted the disease. Unfortunately, Europeans had no immunity to syphilis, and it spread throughout the continent with very serious consequences.

In more recent times, too, brand-new diseases have appeared seemingly out of nowhere. The first case of Legionnaire's disease appeared in 1977, and the first case of AIDS (acquired immune deficiency syndrome) was diagnosed in the United States in 1980.

Why bother to trace the history of a disease at all? Quite often a little piece of information can help define the cause and lead to a cure or effective treatment. While medical debates still continue over the origin of MS, there is convincing evidence that MS was new on the scene in the 1830s.

What We Know about MS Today

Multiple sclerosis is a disease that strikes only the central nervous system, which consists of the brain and spinal cord. These organs control the movements and functions of the entire body. As the brain sends and receives signals, the spinal cord funnels them in and out, to and from different parts of the body through a network of nerves.

The nerves are surrounded by insulating matter called myelin—a soft, white, fatty substance that forms a protective sheath for the nerves. The myelin sheath, which develops in the first ten years of life, insulates the nerve fibers and helps conduct signals through the body.

Multiple sclerosis is a disease where the myelin breaks down and is replaced by scar tissue. This demyelination can slow down or even block the flow of signals to and from the central nervous system to the rest of the body, impairing such functions as vision, strength, or coordination. One important characteristic of myelin, however, is that it can repair itself. This ability, called remyelination, is one of the reasons MS is usually associated with many attacks, or exacerbations, and recoveries, or remissions.

No one knows what actually causes MS, but we do know that it is an acquired disease—you are not born with it. Multiple sclerosis is also an exogenous disease, meaning that it is contracted from the outside. And fortunately, it is not contagious. American researchers have shown that the rate of increased prevalence among husbands and wives is only 1 percent. In England, the prevalence of MS among husbands and wives is less than among the general population, occurring at a rate of 4.9 per 10,000 compared with 5.0 per 10,000.

Multiple sclerosis is often confused with other diseases, most commonly muscular dystrophy (MD) and arteriosclerosis. Multiple sclerosis is not related to either. Muscular dystrophy is a disease of the muscles; arteriosclerosis is a disease that causes hardening of the arteries and blood circulation problems. Because MS is confined to the central nervous system, it has been confused with amyotrophic lateral sclerosis (ALS), also known as Lou Gehrig's disease. Amyotrophic lateral sclerosis is a disease of the nervous system, but it is very different from MS; it has no effect on the myelin sheath but destroys the motor neurons in the central nervous system that directly control muscles.

Who Gets MS?

The focus of much MS research has been in the area of epidemiology—the study of diseases in terms of their geographic and ethnic occurrence, with analysis of all factors including environment and heredity. The epidemiology of MS is nothing less than intriguing.

Prevalence

Since World War II more than 250 prevalence studies of multiple sclerosis have been conducted. As seen in much of the medical literature, many of the studies conflict. According to the National MS Society, the number of reported cases of MS in the United States is approximately 250,000. The actual number of Americans with MS, however, may be closer to 500,000. Because many patients with minor symptoms never consult a doctor about them, they often ascribe the condition to stress, nerves, and other self-diagnosed causes. Additionally, with recent technological advances, the number of MS cases may climb even higher. New diagnostic tools are showing that many people have "silent" MS: They have MS lesions throughout their central nervous systems, but they never have a single manifestation of the disease.

Age

There is no question that multiple sclerosis has a specific age of onset when symptoms first appear. MS rarely strikes before age ten or after age fifty, and symptoms generally appear between ages twenty and forty. Statistically, the average age of onset is twenty-eight, and the average age of diagnosis is thirty-three. (The average age of onset is slightly lower for women than men.)

Socioeconomic Factors

Interestingly, the richest countries, with the highest standards of sanitation, have the highest incidence of MS. The poorest countries, with lower standards of hygiene, have the lowest percentage of MS cases. Two large and carefully conducted American studies, along with another from England, have shown that MS has a predilection for the socially privileged. The evidence suggests that people in less sanitary communities may develop some sort of immunity to MS early in life. Although other studies from Ireland, Israel, the Canadian city of Winnipeg, and the Orkney Islands off northern Scotland do not support these findings, MS has maintained its reputation as a disease of the middle and upper classes.

Geographical Distribution

Worldwide research shows that MS has a definite geographical distribution. It has been long established that MS is more prominent in colder regions and very rare in subtropical and tropical areas—the farther away from the equator, the higher the incidence of MS. In the United States, the farther north, the more MS. And, in fact, if a line were drawn straight along the thirty-seventh parallel, the incidence above the line would be almost twice that below it: Canada has twice the MS incidence of the United States.

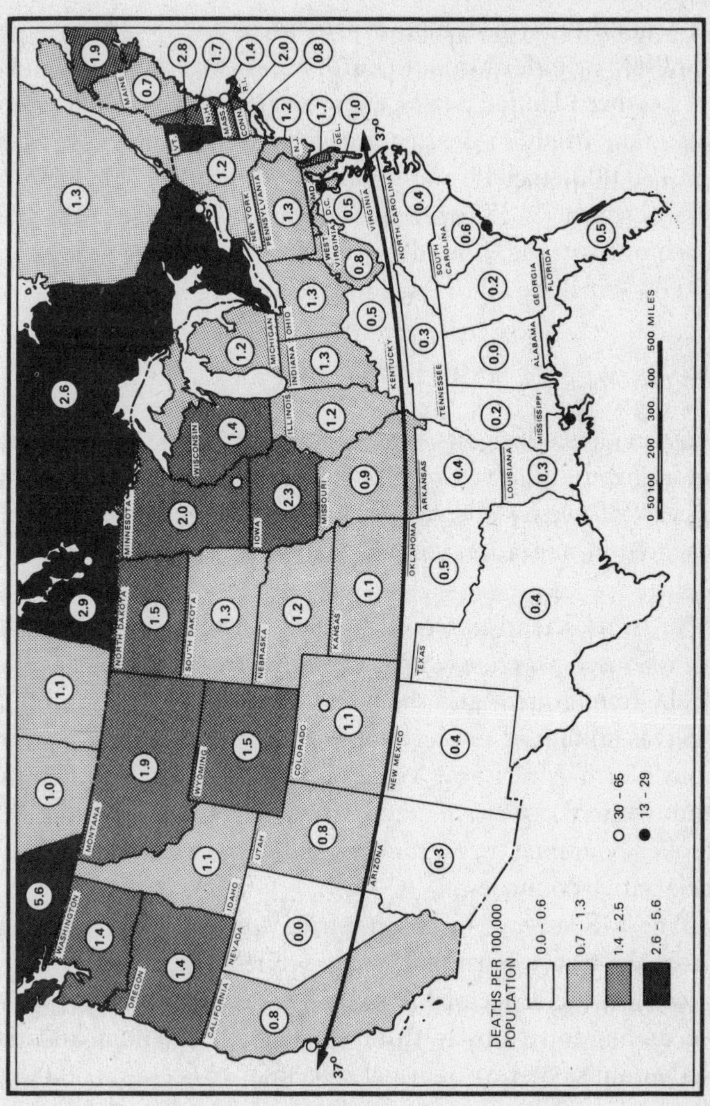

Distribution of MS in the United States.
(Courtesy Louis J. Rosner)

Around the world, high-density areas of MS (30 cases per 100,000) include northern Europe into the USSR, Canada, the northern United States, New Zealand, and southeastern Australia. Medium-density areas (between 5 and 29 cases per 100,000) include nothernmost Scandinavia, the central USSR, southern Europe, the southern United States, and much of Australia. Low-density areas (fewer than 5 cases per 100,000) include all of Asia and the tropics.

Migration

Most evidence suggests that exposure to MS occurs before age eighteen, followed by a latency period (before symptoms appear) of twenty-one years. This has been most clearly documented in migration studies conducted in Israel and South Africa.

In Israel scientists recorded every single case of MS—the age of onset, where each patient came from, at what age he or she immigrated, and the latency period. They found that MS was unknown among native-born sabras and immigrants from North Africa and Yemen but high among immigrants from western, northern, and eastern Europe. In fact, the MS frequency among immigrants matched the incidence rates in their native countries.

The MS surveys in South Africa were equally revealing. There the native-born blacks and whites were found to have a very low incidence of MS (only 3 cases per 100,000), while the immigrants, mostly from the United Kingdom and the Netherlands, had a high incidence (50 cases per 100,000). However, studies also showed that when northern Europeans immigrated before age fifteen, they had the same lowered risk of MS as did native South Africans.

Both the Israeli and South African studies suggest that immigrants with MS were exposed to the inciting agent in childhood and developed symptoms many years later. But what were they exposed to in those crucial years? Something in the soil or the water? Or could it be the climate? Hot or cold weather doesn't cause a disease, but it can certainly have an effect on other aspects of life, such as home heating and ventilation, how much time is spent indoors, and what types of food are eaten.

A truly interesting study just published in the December 20, 2006 issue of the *Journal of the American Medical Association* added to the growing body of evidence that shows that a form of vitamin D may put one at lower risk for developing MS. Researchers looked at a 7 million person database of active-duty military personnel and found the risk of developing MS decreased with higher serum levels of 25-hydroxyvitamin D, the vitamin D that comes with exposure to sunlight and ultraviolet light, rather than from food. (Taking excessive vitamin D supplements can have serious, toxic effects on the body.) This study certainly can help explain the low incidence of MS nearer to the equator, where exposure to ultraviolet light is greatest. And, the study suggests, further research might now examine if vitamin D can alter the course of MS once it has started.

Race

Certain racial groups actually get no MS at all. They are the Eskimos, the Gypsies, the Yakuts in Siberia, and the Bantu in Africa. Among other black groups in Africa, MS is rare. In America blacks have about half the incidence of MS as does the white population. In England blacks also have a much lower incidence than whites. In London a prevalence study was done on black immigrants from the West Indies. More than one hundred cases were predicted for this population, but only eleven cases were ever observed. In the United States black veterans were found to have a 0.4 percent relative risk compared to that of white veterans. MS is more common, however, among American blacks than it is among African and Caribbean blacks—a factor possibly arising from environmental factors or reflecting interracial ancestry.

Many Asian groups in the United States, such as the Japanese and Chinese, have a very low incidence of MS—calculated as low as one-tenth that of many neighboring white populations. The Japanese are probably the most-studied Asian population in regard to MS. While the disease is very rare in Japan, it is equally rare in Japanese who immigrate into other countries. In Los Angeles, where the risk of MS is moderate, and Seattle, where it is high, MS remains very rare among the Japanese populations, even among those locally born. These findings lend credence to the theory that some people can have a genetic insusceptibility to MS.

Although the data are not abundant, it also appears that MS is less common among North American Indians, some Indian groups in South America, and among people born in India, Pakistan, Sri Lanka, and Malta.

Sex

Surveys of patients all over the world show that more women than men get multiple sclerosis. Two separate studies in the United States reported a female-to-male ratio of 1.8 to 1. A survey in western Australia reported a 2.8 to 1 ratio of women to men; and among those born in South Africa, a female-to-male ratio of 2.5 to 1 is accepted. One broader-based study that actually reviewed fourteen different surveys concluded that the average risk for women as compared to men was 1.4 to 1.

Which survey should be accepted? Perhaps none. Taken on face value, they seem to indicate that MS has a definite preference for women, but other factors must be considered. At great risk of sounding sexist, it is our belief that women, in general, pay more attention to their health and see their doctors much more often than do men. So, although surveys show that more women than men contract MS, it is possible that the statistics are weighted in their favor simply because they make themselves more available for neurological assessments.

What Causes MS?

Cruveilhier's original descriptions in the nineteenth century attributed the disease to the suppression of sweat. That theory has long been abandoned, but since then there has been endless speculation as to what causes MS. Some present-day theories are increasingly convincing. But a long process of elimination has narrowed down the field to a few possible causes.

At this point in medical history, scientists acknowledge eleven basic causes of all disease. Every disease known to man is caused by something:

1. Toxic
2. Vascular
3. Metabolic
4. Hereditary
5. Congenital
6. Degenerative
7. Psychogenic

or by:

8. Tumors
9. Trauma

10. Infection
11. Allergy

Each one of the eleven basic causes of disease has been scrutinized for MS. Here is how scientists over the last century have pushed closer and closer to pinpointing its cause.

Toxic

Because of the unique geographical distribution of MS, scientists were naturally drawn to the idea that a toxic agent might cause the disease. Over the decades they have studied soil and water to see if the disease might be related to an excessive content of such minerals as aluminum, copper, manganese, and others. But the enormous variety of toxic elements across latitudes spanning four continents led scientists to rule out a geological factor. Toxins in the diet, even the air, were also evaluated. For instance, high gluten foods such as wheat were once thought to be the possible culprit. But completely removing gluten from the diet did nothing to alter MS statistics. To date, all toxic elements that have been studied, including cosmic rays in the atmosphere, have been ruled out as the cause of MS.

Probably the best argument against a toxic theory comes from studies of an MS "epidemic" in the Faeroe Islands. The Faeroes are a group of fifteen volcanic islands between Iceland and Scotland. Before 1943 not a single case of multiple sclerosis had been discovered among the native Faeroese. Then, between 1944 and 1949, the average annual incidence rate rose to 7.1 cases per 100,000. There is little question among scientists that this development was directly related to the between 1,500 and 7,000 British troops who were stationed in the Faeroes for five years beginning on April 13, 1941.

Investigators believe that British troops, who were carriers of an infectious agent but without symptoms, brought MS to the islands.

If the British troops had introduced multiple sclerosis to the islands by introducing a toxin, MS would still be around. But this is not the case. Instead, the disease almost disappeared with the evacuation of the British forces. Two later "epidemics" were attributed to the Faeroese, who were now carriers themselves, but manifested no symptoms.

Although the studies of the Faeroes ruled out a toxic theory, other important conclusions were drawn. These included the following key points:

1. MS is a unique, widespread, specific infectious disease that only rarely causes symptoms.
2. Acquisition will take place at the first sufficient exposure between ages eleven and forty-five.
3. The disease remains systemic, or in the body, but causing no damage. Subsequently it either invades the nervous system or disappears.
4. It may be transmissible from person to person but only during part or all of the systemic phase.

In conclusion, no toxic-agent theory has ever held up under scientific scrutiny. But, even with lack of evidence, it may still be possible that some toxic agent not yet proposed is the cause of MS.

Vascular

Long ago, doctors suspected that MS was caused by something vascular, or related to the blood circulation. The key theory was that something was wrong with the blood vessels, that myelin lesions were possibly caused by spasms of the arteries. As medical technology progressed and tests such as the angiogram could actually examine blood vessels, doctors were able to see that MS patients had perfectly normal vascular systems.

Metabolic

A metabolic disease would reflect some internal chemical abnormality in the body—such as a disturbance of hormones, sugar levels, or enzymes. Because the age of onset in women is closely associated with puberty, and the risk of developing MS decreases around the time of menopause, scientists examined a hormonal association. But when no hormonal changes were consistently found in MS patients, this association was soon ruled out. At one time MS was also blamed on high blood sugar. Twenty years ago, a neurology resident gave a diabetes drug called Orinase to an MS patient. (Orinase was also being used at the time to treat acne.) Incredibly, the man's MS went into remission. The resident then gave Orinase to seven other patients who allegedly went into remission, too. After this was published in the highly regarded *Journal of the American Medical Association,* MS clinics across the country tested very large groups, unfortunately without any scientific benefits. Similarly, other metabolic causes have been considered and rejected. These include dietary and nutritional theories about both excesses and deficiencies.

Hereditary

In July 2007 prominent scientists announced a true breakthrough in genetics: They identified two genes conclusively linked to MS, the first discovered in over twenty years. Teams of international researchers scanned the human genome of more than 12,000 people of MS risk factors and uncovered the two genes suspected to have a role in autoimmune disease. Until this report, the only genetic link to MS was a large cluster of genes called the major histocompatibility complex (MHC). Now scientists are looking at interleuken-7, or IL-7 receptor and interleuken-2, the IL-2 receptor. IL-7 helps regulate T cells; IL-2 has been linked to type 1 diabetes and autoimmune thyroid disease.

"Having this genetic road map will be of incredible importance in developing new therapies," said Dr. David Hafler of Harvard Medical School, who worked on the genome study. "The study here is the commonality of autoimmune disease," he added.

Still, researchers believe both genetic and environmental factors play a role in developing MS. There is interesting evidence of a slight increase in MS among first-degree relatives—parents, siblings, and children. One recent extensive study (Sadovnick and Macleod, 1981), in British Columbia, ascertained a risk factor of from 1 to 3 percent. Other studies show as much as a 4 percent increase in MS among siblings. This slight increase over the general population is attributed to the greater likelihood of common exposure to whatever the mystery MS element may be. If MS is caused by something in the environment such as a virus (as many scientists suspect), there's a good chance that brothers and sisters are exposed together while growing up. They play in the same school yard, walk the same dog, eat the same foods, breathe the same air, and pass each other the same cold, flu, and measles viruses.

It is also suspected that some family members may even inherit a genetic susceptibility to MS. This is suspected in other diseases, too. For example, if two people each smoke three packs of cigarettes a day, why does one get lung cancer and the other not? A genetic susceptibility is one likely explanation.

A Canadian study of twins published in the *New England Journal of Medicine* (December 1986) has provided the strongest evidence yet of a genetic link for MS. The study found that in nearly 26 percent of identical twins studied both had MS if one did, while in only 2.3 percent of fraternal twins both had the disease if one did. This was a very significant finding, since identical twins come from a single egg and share all their genes, while fraternal twins come from separate eggs and have different genes. The study also showed that in some cases, the "healthy" identical twin had MS lesions, although the disease had never caused symptoms.

In the last ten years, researchers have found that the white blood cells of some people with MS have different human leukocyte antigens (HLA) than those of people without the disease. The HLA system is thought to be connected to the genes that control the immune system. The patterns of these antigens are inherited and can be traced much like blood types.

In the United States and northern Europe, three different HLA antigens are found in higher levels in people with MS than in those without the disease. MS populations in other parts of the world test higher for other HLA antigens. Obviously, the push is on to find if there is one HLA antigen found in the white blood cells of all people with MS and absent from all those without it. When and if this happens, the "susceptibility gene" will have been discovered.

While it is possible to inherit a genetic susceptibility to MS, it is not possible to inherit the disease. And even people who have all the necessary genes don't necessarily get MS.

The disease, experts believe, must be triggered by environmental factors.

For MS to be considered a hereditary disease, the percentage of cases among all siblings, not just identical twins, would have to be 25 percent or more. Since it is not, in spite of the suspected genetic link, MS is not considered a hereditary disease.

Congenital

A congenital disease is one with which a person is born. But since there has never been any evidence that people are born with faulty myelin, congenital theories have basically been ruled out. If people were born with faulty myelin, it wouldn't take so long to show up. The cause for MS must account for its age of onset.

Degenerative

This is a category of disease in which degeneration occurs in a part of the body due to an unknown cause. An example of a degenerative disease is Alzheimer's, in which brain cells begin to die off for no apparent reason. Although *degenerative* is a scientifically accepted category, it is basically a wastebasket category for the incurable diseases that have no known cause. MS was once in this category, but an overwhelming amount of evidence now points to the probability that MS is caused by infection or allergy.

Psychogenic

A psychogenic disease is one that is caused by an emotional condition or process, such as a skin rash or tension headache caused by stress. Although stress, depression, and other emotional factors can aggravate MS, studies show that they do not cause it.

Tumors

Tumors have never been found to cause demyelination and therefore have never been suspected of causing MS.

Trauma

At one time, trauma, or injury, was thought to be the cause of MS. This was based on anecdotal accounts, not scientific evidence. Doctors still see many cases in which a patient has a minor injury, such as stubbing a toe in the middle of the night, and wakes up the next morning with numbness in the entire leg. But since this happens on very rare occasions, scientists consider trauma to be a precipitator of an MS attack rather than a cause of the disease.

Infection

From the start, infection, whether bacterial or viral, has been a strong suspect as the cause of MS. At one time tuberculosis (TB), a disease caused by a bacterium, was linked to MS. But since TB has been drastically reduced and MS is still around in stable numbers, we know there is no correlation.

Spirochetes, spiral-shaped bacteria, were another area of investigation. Since one kind of spirochete causes syphilis, a disease that also produces spotty lesions, it was a reasonable hunch. But studies showed no link to MS there, either; other bacterial leads also failed.

Today one of the most popular scientific theories is that MS is caused by viral infection. Actually, for the past one hundred years, scientists have suspected that MS is caused by a virus attack. Charcot's student and successor, Pierre Marie, first raised the possibility in 1884, and today many researchers still believe that a viral hypothesis can best explain the results of many MS studies. In other words, the viral theory seems to fit the other pieces of the MS puzzle.

The word *virus* comes from the Latin for "slimy liquid," "stench," or "poison." Most of us are familiar with acute viral diseases—such as the flu, a cold, or pneumonia—that hit and leave fairly quickly. These are not caused by the kind of viruses linked to MS. Research is pointing to "slow-acting viruses" that can stay inside the body for months or years before triggering illness. Three areas of investigation have given credence to this theory:

1. Migration studies indicate that MS is related primarily to environmental exposure in childhood followed by a long latency.
2. Animal studies have documented that viruses can evoke relapsing and remitting courses (often seen in MS) and can cause myelin destruction.
3. Studies of MS patients have consistently shown abnormal levels of viral antibodies, the substances the body produces to fight infection.

If a specific virus causes MS, it has yet to be found. At one time or another almost every virus has been investigated for MS, but research in this area still continues. Since 1946 twenty viruses have been studied, and in eleven, high antibody titers (strengths) have been found in the spinal fluid of people with MS. One of the most scrutinized is rubeola, the virus that causes measles.

Rubeola also causes another neurological disease called subacute sclerosing panencephalitis (SSPE)—a slowly progressive disease that occurs as a complication after measles but many years later. In SSPE, antibody levels against the measles virus are unusually high, and there is also demyelination.

The obvious question in early research was, If the rubeola virus could cause SSPE, could it cause MS? The plot thickened in 1962, when Adams and Imagawa reported that antibodies against the measles virus were present in the spinal fluid of more than 75 percent of MS patients and absent in the control group. More than thirty other studies confirmed these findings.

The age factor added one more interesting dimension. In three case-controlled surveys, the MS group had a history of measles at an older age (eleven to fifteen) than the general population. This is particularly intriguing since those who acquired SSPE had measles before age two.

As may be imagined, measles has been studied and studied, but unfortunately, MS researchers have only been able to show a circumstantial association. Other reports threw a monkey wrench into the theory. Scientists reported at least four people with MS with no history of measles and no anti-measles antibody.

Scientists looking further into the MS-measles connection hit another dead end when they saw that MS lesions had little resemblance to the damage done by measles in SSPE. Finally, they learned through autopsy studies that although the measles virus is found in the brains of those with SSPE, it has never been found in the brains of MS patients.

For these and other reasons, the measles theory eventually fell by the wayside. But for those who still believe that some relationship exists between MS and measles, there will be a definite answer soon enough. An entire generation of American children has now been vaccinated against rubeola. These children will soon be coming of MS age, and if rubeola is the cause, a dramatic decline and even eradication of MS in the United States should take place very shortly.

It is also possible that MS may be caused or triggered by more than one virus. Studies have already shown high levels of measles antibodies in the spinal fluid of MS patients. Additional studies have found even higher levels of antibodies against other viruses, including herpes simplex, influenza C, Epstein-Barr, and others. In one study, 23 percent of MS patients had abnormal levels of antibodies to two or more viruses. In 1985 researchers at the Wistar Institute in Philadelphia implicated a new retrovirus, human T-cell lymphotropic virus I (HTLV-I), in as many as one-third of people with MS. A retrovirus is a type of virus that invades a cell and, through a very complex process called "reverse transcription," can produce unlimited copies of itself. Japanese scientists also found antibodies for the HTLV-I virus in the blood of eleven out of forty-six people with MS. This report caused a great deal of concern among patients who feared that the HTLV-I virus might somehow be connected to the HTLV-III virus, which causes AIDS. It is not. There is no AIDS-MS connection at all.

Further studies still have to be conducted to see if HTLV-I is really unique to MS or if it is also found in people with other neurological diseases. Although each new report is interesting, each must be greeted with caution. In 1982, for instance, scientists claimed the subacute myelo-optic neuropathy (SMON) virus was present in the spinal fluid of people with MS. Soon after, however, this "virus" was also found in the spinal fluid of people with illnesses unrelated to MS. The connection between HTLV-I and MS remains to be drawn scientifically. Until then, it must be considered casual.

If multiple sclerosis *is* caused by a virus, how is it contracted?

Viral infections can be divided into three groups: (1) those transmitted by insects such as mosquitoes, ticks, or biting flies; (2) those transmitted by exposure to or consumption of animals that are host to the virus; and (3) those transmitted from human to human.

Insects

Although insects can transmit viruses to humans, it is highly unlikely that MS is transmitted this way. All of the known insect-transmitted diseases, such as encephalitis and yellow fever, are acute virus infections without the latent nature of MS.

Exposure to or Consumption of Animal Carriers

Some of the most emotional arguments concerning MS center around the theory that the disease may possibly be transmitted by dogs and that the virus that causes MS might be canine distemper. Canine distemper is caused by a virus related to measles. It is an acute respiratory and gastrointestinal disease often complicated by a central nervous system disorder that can occur weeks or months later.

It has been proposed that exposure to the canine distemper virus (CDV) or exposure combined with, perhaps, a faulty measles immunity might cause MS. Although these theories rank among the most controversial, they do shed some light on some of the more peculiar MS clusters. One of the most intensively studied is in the Orkney Islands off the northeastern coast of Scotland. In contrast to the Faeroe Islands, which had one major epidemic, the Orkneys have consistently had the world's highest MS rate for the past century. (Prevalence rates have been as high as 309 per 100,000 compared with 58 per 100,000 in the United States today.) Oddly, it was recently discovered that MS incidence rates in the Orkneys have fallen significantly. In the most recent survey, taken on September 21, 1983, the prevalence rate had dropped to 193 per 100,000.

According to published research (*Neurology,* April 1985),

the decline of MS in the Orkney Islands is linked to the decline of CDV, which until 1959 was "frequent, severe, and widespread." And, as in the Faeroes, British troops were stationed there during World War II. Veterinarians in the Orkneys reported that as the troops increased (ultimately to 60,000), so did the dog population. Puppies born on farms all across the islands were taken in as pets. It is believed that when the soldiers left, they left their dogs behind, and large numbers of strays roamed the deserted camps. Although CDV was always prevalent before the war, it became much more severe with the increase in the dog population.

Could this also explain the epidemic in the Faeroes? Did the presence of British troops cause an increase in the dog population and subsequent CDV incidence? Proponents of the CDV-MS hypothesis argue a strong connection.

Researchers have also used the CDV-MS hypothesis to explain an MS "time cluster" in Iceland following widespread CDV epidemics in 1921 and 1941. Ten years after each CDV epidemic, the annual incidence of MS increased significantly.

Why, then, does the CDV theory remain so controversial? Because most surveys have failed to show that people with MS include more dog owners or people who have had greater exposure to dogs. Another criticism of the theory is that while MS has a preference for colder climates, CDV occurs everywhere. (On the other hand, some argue, distemper peaks in cold, damp weather conditions, when dogs and people are more apt to be indoors and in close contact, and CDV is also more rapidly inactivated in warm temperatures.)

As the controversy continues, both sides agree to err on the side of caution and make sure dogs are vaccinated against distemper.

Human to Human

Most likely, MS is not transmitted from human to human. If it were, the number of cases would have reached outrageously epidemic proportions. The low incidence of MS among married couples establishes that it is definitely not transmitted from adult to adult. But can it be transmitted from human to human during the vulnerable years? There is very strong evidence against this theory, but like many theories in MS research, it has not been absolutely ruled out. If MS is, indeed, caused by a virus, exposure to it occurs in one of the three ways just explored.

Allergy

The last consideration is allergy. This would not be an allergy to an environmental substance such as a hay fever attack from pollen or a skin rash from a new soap. What scientists link to this disease is *autoimmunity*—when a person becomes allergic to his or her own tissue and produces antibodies that attack healthy cells.

A well-known example of an autoallergy is rheumatic fever, in which the person's own antibodies attack heart valves and joints. Rheumatic fever actually starts with a streptococcus infection (such as strep throat in childhood). The individual produces antibodies against the infection, but later, those antibodies backfire and attack healthy tissues by mistake. This is called an autoimmune reaction.

There are many autoimmune diseases such as rheumatoid arthritis (in which antibodies attack joints), lupus (in which antibodies attack small blood vessels), and myasthenia gravis (in which antibodies attack muscles).

There is very strong evidence that multiple sclerosis is an autoimmune disease in which the body's own defense system mistakenly forms antibodies that attack myelin. Three areas of research support this theory. First, in laboratory animal experiments, scientists have been able to produce antibodies that attack myelin, so they know it is possible. Second, it has been known for fifty-five years that the spinal fluid of people with MS shows an increased level of antibodies called immunoglobulins. And third, treatments directed against the autoimmune process are often effective.

In summary, it seems very likely that the initial event that starts MS is a viral infection, but the autoimmune process is what keeps MS going.

To date, no specific antibody for multiple sclerosis has been identified, and attempts to show response to brain or viral material have failed. So, while all the abnormalities are intriguing, there is no scientific proof as yet. Still, the combination theory of an early virus attack causing a later autoimmune response is, many believe, the most logical explanation.

2

Symptoms and Signs

Clinically, the hallmark of MS is the attack—the rapid appearance over a week or two of new symptoms that usually last two to six weeks but sometimes six months or more. Attacks vary greatly from person to person and from time to time in the same person. While some patients experience a combination of symptoms all at once, others find they appear one at a time. In some cases, patients have MS with no symptoms at all.

A description of the clinical picture of MS includes *symptoms,* the patient's complaints, and *signs,* what the doctor finds in an examination, such as a change in the knee-jerk reflex test. Together, they are called "findings" and are the principal clues to accurate diagnosis and eventual prognosis.

Symptoms and signs are most commonly believed to be the result of MS lesions causing disturbances in electrical conduction in one or more of three general sites in the central nervous system—the optic nerve, the brain stem–cerebellum, and the spinal cord. As each area controls particular functions of the central nervous system, the location of the lesion will determine the type of attack. For example, an optic nerve lesion may cause blurred vision, blind spots, or a decrease in brightness. A brain stem–cerebellar lesion can cause dizziness or double vision or balance and coordination trouble. Spinal cord lesions give rise to symptoms such as weakness or numbness of the limbs. Occasionally, signs and symptoms are caused by lesions in a fourth area, the cerebrum. This area, however, remains something of a puzzle. Although the pathological lesions of MS are very common there, cerebral signs and symptoms are relatively rare. This discrepancy between lesions and clinical signs and symptoms is one of the great curiosities of MS; many, possibly most, MS plaques are "silent." In fact, a January 1986 study at the Neurologic Institute of the Millard Fillmore Hospital in Buffalo, New York, found that 75 percent of all lesions were "clinically silent."

Why do only a few plaques produce the symptoms and signs? After 100 years, researchers are only beginning to understand. It is now believed that demyelination, even in a large lesion, may have occurred slowly, involving only a small percentage of the fibers that make up the sheath. If remyelination has also occurred, conduction of brain signals to the body can still be maintained. Conduction may be slowed, as specialized tests can reveal, but the patient feels normal.

When MS is not silent in the central nervous system, individuals will face the appearance and disappearance of various signs and symptoms. Although some are common and some very rare, all are important to understand. A basic knowledge of the clinical features of MS is the first step in taking control. It's not only vital for proper diagnosis, but for therapy and management, too. Still, the process of learning about each clinical feature of MS can be trying, especially as you begin to read about some of the less pleasant things that can possibly happen in the course of the disease. It's easy to become overwhelmed and, with each new medical detail, to start to wonder which symptom you'll get and which symptom might get you. The avid jogger worries that her future symptoms will interfere with her running. The pianist panics that his next attack will ruin his finger dexterity. The copy editor is sure she's targeted for blurry vision. At this point, a keen imagination can go into overdrive. And, in this respect, MS patients and sophomore medical students have a lot in common. Both often "develop" many of the ailments they study. Friends and relatives reading about MS symptoms are also not immune. For example, everyone has experienced the feeling of "pins and needles" in a foot that has fallen asleep. A possible symptom of MS, yes, but certainly not a reason to yell, "Aha, it's happening to me, too!" It's much more likely to be the result of sitting in a cramped position too long.

As you read the list of MS symptoms and signs, do not be dismayed. Keep in mind that no two patients have the same symptoms in the same way. MS attacks fall into four patterns that simplify the description of the disorder. Most attacks will have the features of only one of these patterns—the spinal cord attack, the brain stem–cerebellar attack, the optic nerve attack, or the cerebral attack. No one develops all these symptoms; most people will have only six or seven symptoms throughout the course of the disease. And take comfort in knowing that each and every symptom can remit completely, leaving no residual damage. Dramatic recoveries occur from even the worst attacks. Many of the symptoms described may have a simple explanation other than MS. Numbness, tingling, weakness, stiffness, urinary frequency, unsteadiness, incoordination, slurred speech, and blurred vision may each be due to some other disturbance, including some that are insignificant. Do not assume that every new symptom is a symptom of MS—let the doctor decide. And remember, this chapter represents the *possible* situation a patient *may* or *may not* encounter throughout the entire course of the disease.

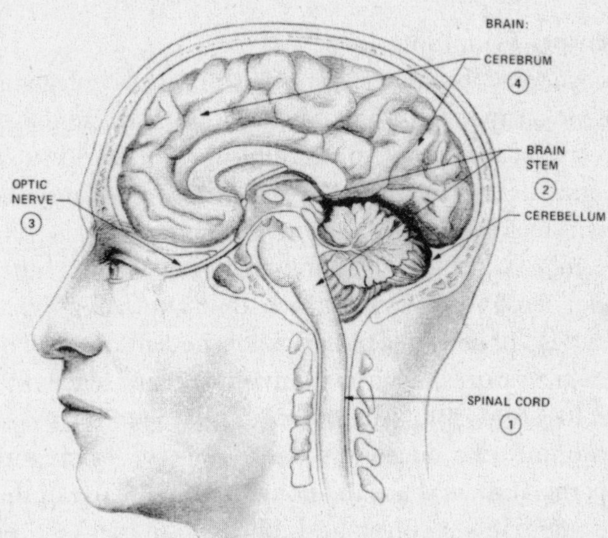

The four areas of the central nervous system that correlate with the symptoms and signs of MS are depicted above and numbered in accordance with the frequency of occurrence of attacks: (1) spinal cord, 42 percent; (2) brain stem and cerebellum, 38 percent; (3) optic nerve, 17 percent; and (4) cerebrum, 3 percent.
(Courtesy Louis J. Rosner/Shelley Ross)

MS Symptoms

Spinal Cord Attacks

The spinal cord attack is the most common type of attack, making up about 42 percent of MS episodes. In this situation the symptoms occur below the neck and fall into two categories—sensory and motor.

Sensory Symptoms

Sensory symptoms consist of disturbances in feeling in the limbs or on the trunk. Symptoms occur because the sensory pathways in the spinal cord are blocked. These disturbances may include one or more of the following: numbness, unpleasant feelings, and Lhermitte's sign.

Numbness, or loss of feeling, may involve just superficial, or skin, sensation, such as the inability to feel a light touch with a wisp of cotton, a pin prick, or the sensations of hot and cold temperatures. Or it may involve deeper sensibility, such as the loss of position sense, the ability to tell the movement, for example, of a finger or toe up or down. When numbness is superficial there is usually no trouble in the use of the limb. If the numbness involves position sense in the hand or foot, the limb will be clumsy in its use.

Unpleasant feelings, or *paresthesias,* include pins-and-needles or tingling, buzzing, and crawling feelings; hot and burning feelings; wetness; tight-band feelings on the trunk (girdle sensations) or around a limb; or feelings of swelling. Some sensations are more difficult to describe. One patient will describe feelings of extra padding (on the sole of the foot, for example); another will describe the presence of a nonexistent foreign object such as crumpled tissue paper or a bandage. Sometimes there will be a feeling of vibration for no apparent reason. Sometimes the skin can feel as if it's burning or cold, or snowflakes falling on the skin can "feel like needles." These odd symptoms, like many others of MS, can unfortunately be mistaken for those of hysteria.

Lhermitte's sign, named after a French neurologist, is technically a symptom, since it is a sensation the patient describes. Many compare the feeling to a lightninglike electrical sensation, or buzzing feeling, that goes down the back to the arms or legs when the head is bent forward as in a barber's chair. The sensation only lasts a second or two. Bending the neck is generally the cause, but coughing or laughing can also trigger it. MS is the most common cause of Lhermitte's sign, but not the only cause.

It must be said again that numbness and paresthesias can be totally benign symptoms, indicating no neurological disease whatsoever. But if the numbness climbs up the legs or arms onto the trunk and comes to a stop at a particular level, then a neurological problem is definitely suggested.

Motor Symptoms

Motor symptoms consist of disturbances in moving one or more limbs. These movement disturbances may include *weakness* or *spasticity* (the tendency of a limb to become stiff and relax only with difficulty) or both.

Weakness: Weakness may be so mild that the complaint will be that the limb just tires easily or feels heavy. Or the weakness may be such that the limb is difficult to lift. Often the weakness disappears after resting or occurs later in the day when the leg, for example, has been fatigued by a lot of standing and walking. Often the individual notices that the toes of shoes wear out prematurely and walking over rough surfaces such as carpets and unpaved walkways is more difficult than over smooth surfaces. Weakness can also appear in the arms or hands, affecting dexterity and causing handwriting to become less legible. Often, in early or mild cases, it is difficult to detect weakness in the limbs in an ordinary exam. But abnormalities can be found in tests of motor reflexes.

Spasticity: Spasticity (rigidity or stiffness) usually involves only the leg, rarely the arm. Individuals may start to notice they can't walk as quickly, or running to catch a ball seems more difficult. Walking up or down stairs is no longer effortless. The limb may stiffen out or draw up involuntarily at times, causing "charley horses" to occur, especially with changes in position such as getting into bed at night. These spasms are more inconvenient than disabling, although some may result in falling without warning.

Weakness by itself is a symptom that brings up many possible diagnoses, with MS far down on the list. Other conditions to consider include pinched nerves, slipped discs, diabetic neuritis, thyroid disease, or even lead poisoning. Weakness with spasticity is more suggestive of something wrong in the spinal cord, with MS high on the list.

Other Spinal Cord Symptoms

Additional symptoms that may occur in a spinal cord attack but are not common include bowel and bladder difficulties and sexual dysfunction.

Bladder symptoms include hesitancy (slowness in starting urination), increased frequency of urination, urgency (the feeling of having to empty the bladder quickly), retention (inability to empty the bladder completely), or episodic incontinence (lack of control). Bowel symptoms include constipation, urgency, and, rarely, incontinence. Sexual dysfunction can include lack of feeling in the genitals, trouble getting or maintaining an erection, or difficulty achieving orgasm. Interestingly, some men can still ejaculate although they can no longer achieve erection. Women have, on occasion, reported a lack of vaginal secretion.

When these additional symptoms occur, they are often not due to MS. Urinary frequency and urgency, especially when there is burning with urination, may arise from a bladder infection. Constipation frequently reflects bad habits in regard to diet or laxatives. Sexual impotence can be entirely psychological, reflecting depression or anxiety. These symptoms are too often wrongly attributed to MS, so it's important that they be discussed with a doctor to avoid jumping to hasty conclusions.

Brain Stem–Cerebellar Attacks

This type of attack is the second most common, constituting about 38 percent of MS episodes. The cardinal symptoms are the three Charcot discovered in his housekeeper. Today called "Charcot's triad," they include double vision, disturbances of balance and coordination, and speech trouble.

Eye Movement Abnormalities

Double vision, or *diplopia,* is the result of either eye-muscle weakness (*gaze palsy,* or *ophthalmoplegia)* or eye-muscle jerking (*nystagmus,* which Charcot's housekeeper had). When these disturbances occur in mild forms, the patient may notice only blurred vision or overlapping or double images. When the disorder is more marked, the complaint may be that of seeing objects jumping. Double vision is also a common symptom of many other disorders, from alcohol and drug abuse to head injury and inner ear infection. In MS, double vision can also occur when the individual is fatigued.

Imbalance and Incoordination

Disturbances of balance and coordination are called *ataxia.* Balance trouble may be associated with *vertigo,* a type of dizziness in which there is a feeling of spinning, turning, falling, floating, or some other false sense of motion. The individual may also experience nausea. With vertigo, the loss of balance may occur only briefly with changes of position, such as when first standing up to walk. Balance difficulty may be without vertigo and more constant, causing the person to sway, tilt, weave, veer, or stagger when walking. There are dozens of other causes of this symptom including alcohol or drug abuse, head injury, inner ear infection, physical exhaustion, and high or low blood pressure. Balance disturbance must be considered in the context of whatever other symptoms and signs the patient is showing before it can be labeled an MS symptom.

Coordination trouble in the hand or foot is somewhat more diagnostic of MS. The patient may report clumsiness, shakiness, slowness, or disturbance in the rhythm of movement in the use of a limb. *Intention tremor,* another of Charcot's triad, is shaking or wavering when attempting to touch a target. When it is the hand that is involved, fine-skilled actions such as writing and buttoning may be disturbed. When it is the leg that is involved, walking will be disturbed. Conventional tests of coordination, such as walking heel to toe in a straight line, become difficult to perform. Incoordination, of course, may be due to factors other than MS—for example, excessive use of alcohol or coffee, reaction to medication, or just emotional tension or exhaustion.

Speech Disorders

Disturbance of pronunciation or rhythm of speech is the last of Charcot's three signs, called *dysarthria.* It is rare and usually found in the more advanced disease. The pronunciation problem begins with the slurring of certain consonants, causing the person to sound as if he or she has had too much to drink. A problem with speech rhythm causes the individual to speak in a jerky, somewhat explosive fashion. This has been called "scanning speech," because it resembles the school exercise in which a line of poetry is scanned, or accented at the proper syllables.

Slurred speech can be due to a variety of disorders, including alcohol and drug abuse. Scanning speech is more suggestive of MS; it rarely occurs in other diseases.

Facial Nerve Abnormalities

Facial weakness, numbness, spasms, palsy, pain, and *myokymia* (the involuntary rapid flickering of facial muscles) occurring on one side of the face, are all symptoms that are not very common but can be MS-related. Facial weakness can also be due to Bell's palsy, a virus infection of the facial nerve.

Trigeminal Neuralgia

Momentary sharp jabs of electric or lightninglike pain following a nerve root down one side of the face occur in some patients. When the pain follows the trigeminal nerve in the face, it is called *trigeminal neuralgia* (or *tic douloureux* in French). It can be triggered by eating, talking, shaving, washing the face, brushing the teeth, or touching the face at the trigger spot. Trigeminal neuralgia occurs in three areas: (1) forehead and eyeball, (2) cheek and nose, midface, and upper lip, and (3) lower jaw and chin. This symptom, however, is also a symptom of diseases other than MS. (Face pain can also result from minor disorders such as a bad bite.) In fact, only about 3 percent of those with trigeminal neuralgia have MS.

Other Brain Stem–Cerebellar Symptoms

Loss of hearing and ringing in the ear, called *tinnitus,* are very rare in MS and limited to one side only. Swallowing difficulty, or *dysphagia,* is also rare, affecting mainly people with long-standing brain stem trouble. Loss of sense of smell and loss of sense of taste have been reported but are very rare. Loss of sense of smell, for example, was reported in only two cases of MS in a survey by McAlpine, one of the most authoritative names in MS literature.

The MS patient can experience emotional disturbances that may include *euphoria,* an exaggerated cheerfulness or feeling of well-being; emotional *lability,* a tendency to get upset or excited easily; and inappropriate or excessive laughing or crying triggered by trivial things or nothing at all. Since mental changes cannot be observed in controlled studies, the clear picture seen with some other MS symptoms is virtually impossible to obtain. Most researchers admit that there is no way of determining whether depression, for example, is actually caused by MS or is the patient's reaction to coping with the disease.

Psychosis, schizophrenia, and other psychiatric disorders are occasionally seen with MS, but experts believe the diseases are not related in any way. Hysteria—in which patients with only mild symptoms of MS start to believe they have worse symptoms and can become incapacitated by them—is also seen from time to time.

Each of these symptoms may result from something other than MS. Hearing loss and tinnitus most probably reflect local trouble in the ear itself. With swallowing trouble, attention should focus first on the throat rather than the brain. Until recently, emotional problems, memory problems, and cognition were considered to have psychological origins until proved otherwise. They are now known to be affected by MS more commonly than was evident in 1992.

Optic Nerve Attacks

The optic nerve attack, or optic neuritis, is third in frequency of occurrence. About 17 percent of MS attacks are of this type. Optic neuritis (ON) is one of the most clearly defined sensory symptoms in MS. It is also one of the most common symptoms a patient will first notice. When it strikes, the patient can often state the time and place it happens.

The classic case of ON starts with the initial symptom of simple blurred vision. There is usually a sudden *onset*—the medical term for the occurrence of the first symptom. ON commonly occurs in one eye and vision can be described as blurry, foggy, misty, cloudy, fuzzy, or distorted. Usually vision loss is in one central spot, called the *scotoma,* or in the entire eye. When the lesion is in the optic *chiasma,* the point where the two optic nerves meet, vision will be impaired on the outer side of each eye. ON in both eyes simultaneously is rare, but it is not uncommon to have ON occur in one eye and later in the other. Depth perception can also be impaired, and patients will describe difficulties in judging steps or the position of a moving ball in games like tennis, golf, or football. Pain and tenderness with eye movement can be present at some stage and can also be accompanied by headache. As vision begins to improve, an effect called *movement phosphenes* can occur, and the patient will see a bright flash upon eye movement in the dark. The pupils' reaction to light is often affected with ON. While the normal pupil will constrict as a reflex reaction to light, it remains relatively dilated in optic neuritis.

The ON attack will usually reach a peak in a few days. Then there is usually a rather quick recovery within two to six weeks. Sometimes the recovery is slow, and occasionally it is incomplete, leaving decreased visual acuity in the affected eye. When individuals do suffer some loss of vision, it is generally modest, with 20/20 vision becoming 20/30 or 20/40. It is a general rule, however, that good vision returns after the initial attack of ON. Nevertheless, complete recovery does not mean that the optic nerve is completely normal, as seen with what is called *Uhthoff's phenomenon.*

Uhthoff's phenomenon was first described in 1890, when the German ophthalmologist Wilhelm Uhthoff discovered that some individuals had temporary blurring of vision following strenuous exercise. Uhthoff's phenomenon usually improves slowly, and most people learn to avoid it. It is thought to be a result of a rise in body temperature.

There are many other possible causes of ON besides MS. These include sinus disease, alcoholism, severe vitamin deficiency, pernicious anemia, diabetes, heavy metal poisoning, autoimmune diseases affecting the vascular system, syphilis, and adverse reactions to vaccination or certain medications such as birth control pills. ON does not always mean MS. And visual symptoms do not necessarily mean optic neuritis. Minor conditions such as eyestrain, overuse of eye drops, eye infections, and blows to the head may be responsible for blurring of vision. It is generally accepted, however, that in the absence of any other cause, ON is probably due to multiple sclerosis.

It's interesting to note that ON is even more common in other parts of the world. In the United States it is an MS symptom in about 18 percent of cases. But a recent onset study revealed that the frequency of ON in Great Britain was 25 percent in one eye and 3 percent in both eyes. The frequency of ON onset in Japan was 48 percent in one eye and 22 percent in both.

Cerebral Attacks

The cerebral attack is a type of episode that rarely occurs in MS, with only a 3 percent incidence rate. The symptoms come on like those of a stroke and include mental disturbance; seizures; loss of speech expression or comprehension *(aphasia);* one-sided visual field loss *(hemianopsia);* or sensory loss or weakness of the face, arm, and leg on one side *(hemiparesis).* Epileptic seizures are occasionally seen with MS, but the conditions are not necessarily related.

In general, cerebral attacks are so unusual in MS that other diagnoses tend to be uppermost in the doctor's thinking until the rapid and complete recovery brings multiple sclerosis to mind.

Transient Attacks

Tonic Seizures

There is a rare phenomenon in MS called the tonic seizure, which is a brief attack, lasting just seconds, in which one side of the body stiffens into a twisted position when the individual gets up to walk. The arm draws up and the leg straightens out. This lasts a few seconds, then the limbs relax and the person can walk. These are not epileptic seizures, however, and the patient remains alert. Tonic seizures are rare, occurring in only 5 out of 800 patients seen by this author.

Paroxysmal Symptoms

When a symptom occurs in brief episodes of a few minutes at a time, it is called a *paroxysm.* Most common are double vision, slurred speech, incoordination, and tonic seizures. *Akinesia,* the inability to move one or more limbs, is another MS paroxysm, although it is more typically a symptom of Parkinson's disease. Paroxysmal symptoms, sometimes lasting only twenty seconds, usually remit and relapse just as in other MS attacks. Symptoms appear suddenly and continue with a degree of intensity, then remit completely after a few days or weeks.

Fatigue

Fatigue is a symptom of MS that's in a category of its own since it cannot be traced to any one spot in the nervous system. While it is the single most common complaint of patients, it is also the one symptom to which others are least sympathetic. Especially in the absence of other symptoms, others can easily regard it as laziness, depression, or copping out. This is unfortunate because, although fatigue is invisible, it can often be the most debilitating of symptoms.

There is not yet a good anatomical explanation for the fatigue of MS. Sometimes it is due to subtle weakness in the legs. Sometimes it is the result of the extra work required to stay active in spite of a balance or coordination problem. Sometimes it is related just to the frustration of having MS. In any case, fatigue often occurs in isolation, unassociated with other symptoms, when the MS has gone into remission.

Fatigue commonly strikes in the late afternoon, when the body temperature normally rises. Frequently fatigue is relieved by cooling off and resting. By early evening, when the body temperature starts to fall again, fatigue will subside.

Fatigue, though very real and sometimes very debilitating, is one of the more deceptive complaints of MS. Patients can look terrific but feel exhausted. This is one reason why collecting disability insurance for fatigue has been a controversial issue.

MS Signs

Before long, the patient experiencing neurological symptoms will wind up in the office of a neurologist, a physician who specializes in the nervous system. The neurologist will conduct a neurological examination to search for clues. Here is a breakdown of what the doctor is looking for and what each abnormality means.

Mental State and Speech

While talking with the patient, the doctor is also evaluating the individual's mental state, noting especially the presence of emotional lability. At the same time, speech will be evaluated. The patient may later be asked to repeat certain standard phrases that may reveal problems with enunciation and rhythm. Slurring of speech and scanning speech are the important things to note, since they may indicate a brain stem–cerebellar lesion.

Eyes

Next is the examination of the eyes. In an optic neuritis attack, the doctor looks for particular findings. Visual acuity, or sharpness, is tested by means of the eye chart. It will be decreased in the affected eye. The fields of vision are tested when the patient is asked to look straight ahead and to indicate when an object comes into view from each side. This may reveal right or left hemianopsia or show an abnormal blind spot (scotoma) in the center of vision or off to the side. The optic nerve is examined by the ophthalmoscope, which enables the doctor to look at the back of the eye. With MS, the optic nerve may appear pale, red, or swollen. Finally, the pupils are checked for appearance and reaction to light and focusing, both close and at a distance.

Eye movements are examined by having the patient look to the right and to the left and up and down. Two abnormalities may be seen that typify MS. One is nystagmus, the involuntary jerking of the eyes as they gaze in different directions or sometimes even at rest. The second is weakness of the eyes, more of one eye than the other, in looking to one side. This asymmetrical gaze weakness is called internuclear ophthalmoplegia. Internuclear ophthalmoplegia indicates a brain stem lesion. Nystagmus points to either the brain stem or cerebellum or their connections to the inner ear.

Two rare signs, which also reveal MS involvement of the brain stem, are third-nervc palsy and Horner's syndrome, both of which show an eyelid droop on one side. In third-nerve palsy, there is also dilation of the pupil and weakness of all eye movements except looking outward. In Horner's syndrome, there is constriction of the pupil and no gaze weakness.

Face, Tongue, and Throat

Testing for sensory loss and weakness in these areas is done by touching with cotton and a pin and by watching the muscles move. Facial movements are also observed as the patient is asked to smile, pucker the lips, puff the cheeks, wrinkle the nose, squeeze the eyes closed, and elevate the eyebrows. The doctor may find sensory loss or weakness on one side of the face, but neither is diagnostic of MS unless combined with other, more typical signs. Numbness and weakness of the back of the throat are tested in two ways: when the patient is asked to say "ah" and when the gag reflex is checked with a tongue depressor. This, along with numbness and weakness of the tongue, is rare in MS and more suggestive of some other disorder.

Hearing

The hearing is tested with a tuning fork at the bone behind the ear and at the outside of the ear opening. Decreased hearing is very rare in MS. Such a finding mandates further tests to rule out other diagnoses.

Sensation

Sensory examination involves the testing of the main parts of the body—face, trunk, arms, and legs—for the modalities of sensation. Sensitivity to touch is tested with a wisp of cotton. Sensitivity to pain is tested with a pinprick. Temperature sensitivity is examined by touching with warm and cold objects. Vibratory sense is tested by placing a vibrating tuning fork on bony prominences. Position sense is tested by having the patient close the eyes and identify upward or downward movements of the fingers and toes. Finally, certain combined sensory modalities are important to examine. *Stereognosis* is the ability to identify, with the eyes closed, common objects such as a coin and a key placed in the hand. Stereognosis requires both normal touch sensation and normal position sense in the hand. The ability to identify two simultaneous touches on the face and hand is called for in *double simultaneous stimulation.* Recognition of whether one or two points are touching the face, hand, or foot is called *two-point discrimination.* Identifying numbers "written" on the palms of the hands is the object of the *palm-writing test.*

Two typical patterns of sensory loss are seen in MS. The first is decreased touch or pinprick sensitivity on the legs and trunk up to a particular level, which may be at the navel, at the bottom of the rib cage, up to the nipple line, or as high as the armpits or neck. The exact upper limit of the level pinpoints the lesion to a particular segment of the spinal cord. The second typical finding is the loss of position sense and stereognosis in the hands. The hands may be normally strong but difficult to use effectively because the patient does not know where the fingers are or what is in the hand without looking. This is called the "useless hands syndrome" and indicates involvement of the cervical (neck) portion of the spinal cord. Frequently, however, the results of the sensory examination are normal in MS, even when the patient is in the midst of a sensory attack.

Motor System

The motor examination includes looking at the muscles for shrinkage *(atrophy),* swelling *(hypertrophy),* and twitching *(fasciculations)*. Muscle tone in the limbs, which may be too loose or too tight, is checked by asking the patient to relax and let each arm and leg be moved back and forth in a swinging motion. Strength in the limbs is tested by having the patient hold the limb against resistance at each joint. Movements at the shoulders, elbows, wrists, hands, hips, knees, ankles, and toes are checked, comparing each side and taking into account the patient's dominant side and general build.

Hand coordination is evaluated by the finger-to-nose test (the patient touches the doctor's finger and own nose) and by the performance of rapid alternating movements (turning the hand over and back, closing and opening the fist in rapid succession, or touching the thumb to each finger up and down the line). Coordination in the leg is evaluated by the heel-knee-shin test, in which the patient is asked to run the right heel down the left shin from knee to ankle and the left heel down the right shin from knee to ankle.

In a spinal cord attack, the doctor may find weakness and increased tone (spasticity) in one or both legs and occasionally in one or both arms. Weakness and spasticity in a limb may also occur with a brain stem or cerebral lesion, but more often in MS, the doctor localizes the trouble to the spinal cord. In a brain stem–cerebellar attack, the findings may include wavering of the finger on the finger-to-nose test (intention tremor), slowness and clumsiness of the hand in doing rapid alternating movements *(dysdiadochokinesis)*, and zigzagging or jerkiness of the foot on the heel-knee-shin test *(dysmetria)*. A limb that shows one or more of these signs of incoordination is said to be ataxic.

Reflexes

Deep tendon reflexes (DTRs) are the involuntary jerks normally produced at certain spots on the limbs by tapping tendons with a reflex hammer. The examination will test for absent, diminished, exaggerated, or asymmetrical reflexes along with "pathological reflexes," which occur in the hand or foot only in abnormal situations. Reflexes commonly tested in the arm are those of the biceps (by tapping at the bend of the elbow), the triceps (by tapping at the back of the elbow), and the radial (by tapping at the side of the wrist). In the leg the reflexes tested include the knee jerk (by tapping below the kneecap) and the ankle jerk (by tapping the back of the heel cord). In the eye the blink reflex is tested by a wisp of cotton or puff of air.

The two most common pathological reflex tests are named for the scientists who discovered them. The Hoffman sign occurs when the middle finger is bent back and flicked, and the thumb and index finger jerk instead of remaining still. The Babinski sign occurs when the sole of the foot is stroked along the side, and the big toe goes up instead of down and the other toes fan out.

In MS, when there is weakness and spasticity in a limb, the reflexes will be increased and a pathological reflex will be present. If there is ataxia in a limb, the reflexes may be decreased. Thus, the relative presence or absence of reflexes serve as confirmatory signs to document a lesion in the spinal cord, brain stem–cerebellum, or cerebrum.

Occasionally, other miscellaneous reflexes are tested in the face, abdomen, and groin. In a normal abdominal reflex the stomach wall twitches when stroked vertically with a stick. If this reflex is diminished, it indicates an abnormal finding. This test, however, is often misleading if the patient has lost reflexes because of such other factors as obesity, abdominal surgery, childbearing, or even too cold a temperature in the examination room. The *cremasteric reflex,* found in males only, is a twitch response that follows the stroking of the inside of the thigh. The absence of this reflex is an abnormal finding. The *palmo-mental sign* is a twitching of the patient's chin when the palm is stroked. Normally there is no reaction. The jaw-jerk reflex occurs when the jaw is tapped while the mouth is open. Normally this test should produce only a slight jerk. It is abnormal when the reflex is more prominent or hyperactive. The snout reflex is tested to see if the lips pout out after the upper lip is tapped while the mouth is closed. Normally there is no response. The *glabellar reflex* is tested to see if the eyes continue to blink after tapping between the eyebrows. Normally the person will blink but stop when the tapping stops. (An abnormal glabellar reflex, however, is more suggestive of Parkinson's disease than MS.) The grasp reflex is tested to check for an involuntary grasp response that occurs when the palm is stroked. Normally the hand remains still. These miscellaneous reflex tests are done on occasion, but the more conventional reflex tests are more valuable and leave less room for subjective observation.

Stance and Gait

Examinations of standing and walking can reveal sensory loss, weakness, spasticity, and ataxia. A patient's stance is tested by having the individual stand with the feet together, arms outstretched in front, and eyes open and then closed. This is called the Romberg test. A person who is having trouble in the balance center of the cerebellum will sway with open eyes. One who has loss of position sense in the feet will sway only with the eyes closed. Other standing tests require the subject to balance on each foot alone and then hop on each foot and march in place with the eyes closed. This may reveal weakness or ataxia in the legs.

In testing gait, the doctor watches the patient walk. Here, arm-swing, leg movement, posture of head and trunk, and straightness of the walk are evaluated. Weakness on one side of the body will be revealed by lack of arm swing and dragging of the leg. Ataxia of trunk or legs will be revealed by staggering or weaving from side to side or by veering or tilting to one side. Position-sense loss in a foot will result in clumsy slapping or slamming of the foot when walking. Other gait tests involve requiring the patient to walk on the toes, walk on the heels, and walk a straight heel-to-toe line (tandem walking). In a spinal cord attack, the patient may drag a leg, slap a foot, or give way with the foot on toe or heel walking. In a brain stem–cerebellar attack, the walk may be unsteady and the tandem walk difficult. These extra tests may also reveal weakness in a foot or subtle ataxia in a leg.

Through such examinations a neurologist may come to suspect MS lesions in the central nervous system, although other problems may also still be under suspicion. At this point the patient and doctor should discuss where the trouble seems to be and what the possible causes are.

MS signs and symptoms can occur with any central nervous system lesion. The frequency of symptoms at onset, according to a five-year study of 253 patients seen by this author at the UCLA Multiple Sclerosis Clinic, is as follows:

1. Sensory	55 percent
2. Ataxia	27 percent
3. Paresis (weakness)	21 percent
4. Optic	18 percent
5. Diplopia	18 percent
6. Vertigo	6 percent
7. Dysarthria	5 percent
8. Facial numbness	4 percent
9. Bladder difficulties	3 percent

10. Lhermitte's sign	2 percent
11. Facial palsy	1 percent
12. Trigeminal neuralgia, girdle sensation	2 patients each
13. Headache, nausea and vomiting, hearing loss and tinnitus, dysphasia, emotional lability	1 patient each

The ten most common symptoms and signs to appear at any time throughout the entire course of MS are:

1. Increase in reflexes	91 percent
2. Ataxia	85 percent
3. Weakness with spasticity	77 percent
4. Sensory loss	75 percent
5. Double vision with nystagmus	65 percent
6. Optic neuritis	53 percent
7. Bladder difficulty	45 percent
8. Slurred or scanning speech	33 percent
9. Gaze weakness	32 percent
10. Vertigo	13 percent

In addition, four phenomena are particularly suggestive of MS:

1. Optic neuritis with scotoma (visual loss with a central blind spot in one eye).
2. Internuclear ophthalmoplegia (asymmetrical gaze weakness).
3. Lhermitte's sign (a sensation of electricity down the back and legs or arms on bending the head).
4. Girdle sensations (tight-band feelings around the trunk).

Before leaving this chapter on symptoms and signs, it's important to remember that no one develops all of these manifestations. In general, patients seen in clinics tend to have more serious symptoms and signs than those seen in private practice. Most people with MS will have only six or seven different symptoms throughout their lives. The pattern of the early attacks will most likely occur in later attacks. All of these symptoms and signs can go away. The large majority of patients will have an episodic course of attacks with remission. Seventy-five percent of people with MS will never need a wheelchair, and 40 percent will experience no interference with normal activity.

Silent MS

In some cases, people who are known to have the lesions of MS have no symptoms throughout their lives. This is called "silent multiple sclerosis." Drs. Markey and Hirano first speculated about silent MS in 1967. More recently, a study suggested that for every four patients clinically diagnosed with MS, there is one person living with silent MS. Independently, at the Basel Institute of Pathological Anatomy in Switzerland, the Georgi series of 15,644 random autopsies found MS lesions in twelve subjects who had no medical history of MS signs or symptoms. Still, there is no answer yet as to why one plaque will cause symptoms and another will not.

3

The Diagnosis

A true revolution has occurred in the diagnosis of MS with the widespread use of magnetic resonance imaging (MRI), which can now show a clear picture of MS lesions in the brain and spinal cord. For years, MS had remained one of the most difficult diseases to confirm. But that has now dramatically changed. But even with the new technology, the diagnostic process is, at best, a complex one, usually beginning with a visit to the family doctor—a general practitioner who is often unprepared for some of the strange descriptions of symptoms. It is not uncommon for a patient to be referred to an ophthalmologist for eye complaints, an orthopedist for problems related to the spine and bones, a urologist for bladder problems, or even a psychiatrist.

In 1879 Dr. Buzzard wrote, "In its infancy, the name we give to multiple sclerosis is hysteria." At the time it was not uncommon for the early signs and symptoms of MS to be confused with psychiatric problems. Today MS remains one of the most difficult diseases in the world to diagnose.

How then is a person ever diagnosed as having MS? Neurologists analyze information in two stages. First they discern where the problem is. Then they must consider what all the causes of disease are in that location. When several locations are involved, the list of possible diagnoses narrows.

To diagnose multiple sclerosis, the neurological evaluation must satisfy two clinical criteria: first, a course of attacks and remissions, and second, findings (either from the neurological examination or the patient's history) that suggest lesions in at least two of the main sites of the central nervous system—spinal cord, brain stem–cerebellum, optic nerve, or cerebrum.

The success of a diagnosis is, of course, highly dependent on the doctor's skill in observing and soliciting an accurate description of history and symptoms. The history begins with the present illness—when and how did it start? It's important to discuss each symptom—if it disappeared and when, if it still persists, if symptoms vary during the day, if it's constant or intermittent, what provides relief, if it's affected by heat from exercise or a hot bath, and so on. Then the patient's past history must be carefully reviewed, taking in any illnesses, injuries, operations, allergies, medications, pregnancies, or alcohol or drug abuse. The neurologist might also take a history from a parent, husband, wife, or other close family member. The family history will include serious medical problems, causes of death, and any other neurological disorders in parents, brothers, sisters, and children. The visit to the neurologist, including the history taking and neurological examination discussed in chapter 2, can take up to two hours. (It should be remembered that the neurologist may also suspect a stroke, a tumor, an adverse reaction to medication, or some other problem.)

Because MS is a disease marked by attacks and remissions, symptoms that appear and disappear, its diagnosis has always been difficult. And even when MS has been strongly suspected, many doctors have often been reluctant to inform the patient of an unconfirmed hunch. Instead, they have been more likely to wait for more signs or symptoms to appear, a process often taking many years. But these are revolutionary times for diagnosticians. Finally, after a century of guesswork and uncertain evaluation, advanced technology allows the first clear visualization of MS lesions. Although there is no actual test to detect the disease, the MRI leaves little doubt in MS diagnoses. The sophisticated $2 million scanners use magnetic fields up to 30,000 times stronger than the earth's radio-wave pulses. These provide pictures of the central nervous system never before seen with X-rays or CAT scanners, the specialized diagnostic tool introduced in the 1970s. The MRI has created a revolution in MS diagnosis.

The MRI has taken much of the guesswork, frustration, and anxiety out of the process. It can almost always confirm a diagnosis. But doctors are still not prescribing them as routinely as dental X-rays. First, the scanners cost approximately $2 million each, plus $1 million more to install. Each scan can run between $1,000 and $1,500, so doctors may choose alternate, less costly laboratory tests early in the elimination process.

Still, the medical community has rallied around the MRI, and for MS patients that's great news. It was only in November 1985 that Medicare agreed to pay for MRI tests. Many private insurance companies, health maintenance organizations (HMOs), and the state Medicaid programs followed. If used properly, all agree, the MRI can actually cut down on hospital costs by cutting down on unnecessary surgery or batteries of unnecessary tests.

LABORATORY TESTS

So what are the other alternative diagnostic tests, and when would you really use them? First, there may not be an MRI in your immediate area. And in some other instances a clear-cut diagnosis still cannot be made with the MRI, a history, and a neurological examination. For instance, the history may suggest MS, but only one lesion may be found. Or another disease must be confirmed or ruled out. Often, depending on the evaluation, the neurologist may suggest one of three categories of laboratory tests for further confirmation: spinal tap, evoked response tests, or imaging of the central nervous system.

Spinal Tap

The spinal tap is a routine diagnostic test that was first performed in 1891. From its beginning, the spinal tap has been the target of a lot of bad press. In reality a spinal tap is a simple, relatively painless procedure done in a doctor's office, an outpatient clinic, or a hospital. After Novocain is administered to the lower back, a needle is inserted and spinal fluid withdrawn. This is done well below where the spinal cord ends, so there is no danger. It is no more traumatic than having blood drawn. But in spite of its benign nature, the average person still views the spinal tap as the one test to fear. This is unfortunate, since various tests on spinal fluid have been very valuable in helping to diagnose MS.

IgG *(immunoglobulin G)* is the substance that represents increased antibody formation. An elevated level in the spinal fluid suggests the presence of an autoimmune phenomenon. Another type of immune abnormality, the *oligoclonal band* (OB), has been picked up in the spinal fluid of as many as 90 percent of MS patients. A third abnormal finding is the presence of a breakdown product of myelin called myelin basic protein (MBP). Until the MRI, identifying these through a spinal tap was as close as it was possible to get to a diagnostic test for MS. But increased IgG can also be seen in other diseases such as encephalitis, lupus, meningitis, and Guillain-Barré syndrome. Oligoclonal bands and myelin basic protein can also be found in other demyelinating diseases besides MS.

Today many neurologists do not feel that these laboratory tests are necessarily the best way to confirm an MS diagnosis. Still, a spinal tap may be necessary if problems other than MS are also suspected, such as an infection in the central nervous system.

Myelogram

In the past, when signs or symptoms were confined to the spinal cord and no dramatic remission occurred, it was frequently necessary to do a myelogram to rule out any compression of the spinal cord by, for example, a disc or tumor. In this test, dye is injected into the spinal fluid and an X-ray is taken. With the MRI, this test is needed much less often.

Evoked Response Tests

An "evoked potential" is the brain's electrical response to stimulation of a sensory system, such as when light is flashed into the eyes. The evoked response test can actually record how long it takes for a stimulus to reach the brain.

Harmless electrodes are attached to the scalp, connecting the patient to a device that records brain waves, called an electroencephalograph (EEG). Three tests are most common: visual, auditory, and pain stimulus.

1. Visual: There are many ways to record visual evoked potentials (VEP), including blink tests and flash responses. The most commonly used visual test is the pattern-shift visual evoked response (PSVEP), which involves a checkerboard pattern flashed in front of the patient's eyes as a computer records the times it takes for the electrical

impulse to reach the visual center in the brain. If the transmission is slow or absent on one side, this confirms an abnormal spot along the visual pathway. The visual evoked response test has proved extremely valuable; it has shown unsuspected lesions in patients who were never even aware of having a visual problem.

2. Auditory: This test records how long it takes for a ten-second click to travel from the ear to the auditory center in the brain. If the response is slow or absent, it frequently indicates the presence of a brain stem lesion. The medical name for this test is the brain stem auditory evoked response (BAER). In a large study of 1,000 MS patients, 46 percent had abnormal BAER results. Other studies show that, in spite of obvious abnormalities, hearing is seldom seriously impaired in MS patients.
3. Pain stimulus: Although visual and sound tests are completely painless, the pain stimulus test (somatosensory evoked potential, or SSEP) can be uncomfortable. It measures how long it takes the brain to record an electrical current on nerves at the finger, wrist, or knee. The SSEP assesses spinal cord and brain stem lesions.

Since part of the diagnostic criteria for MS includes lesions in at least two main sites, the evoked response tests have been very helpful—especially since they can often detect a silent lesion. However, multiple abnormalities on evoked response tests do not categorically point to an MS diagnosis. Vitamin B_{12} deficiency, neurosyphilis, lupus, and other diseases are also known to cause multiple lesions.

Radiology

Until the mid-1970s, radiology consisted primarily of routine X-rays, which have never been useful as a diagnostic tool for

MS. But in 1975 computerized axial tomography, more commonly known as the CAT scan, was first used in the diagnosis of MS. The CAT scan is a sophisticated X-ray technique that takes a picture of a plane in the body both before and after a dye is intravenously injected to enhance the results. Tumors, strokes, atrophy, swellings, and many other disorders never before seen in regular X-rays were now clearly defined. Researchers found that sometimes, if a double dose of dye was used, MS lesions would show up. But this proved to be unreliable.

Then, the magnetic resonance imager (MRI) was introduced to the medical community. The magnetic resonance phenomenon was actually first demonstrated in 1946 by American scientists Edward Purcell and Felix Bloch, who jointly won the Nobel Prize for physics (1952) for their discovery.

The technique has also been called nuclear magnetic resonance (NMR), but the word *nuclear* is misleading to patients. Actually, the magnetic resonance scanner, unlike the X-ray, involves no radiation at all. Instead, the patient is placed in a magnetic field and radio wave pulses are bounced off the body. As this occurs, the MRI measures variations in the energy level of the hydrogen atom nuclei in the cells. No harmful rays are emitted. A harmless dye called Gadolinium is used to enhance the appearance of lesions and to determine if a lesion is new or old. The test is completely safe, effective, and accurate. Patients lie inside a tunnellike machine and while some feel claustrophobic, many fall asleep during the forty-five minute test. As the radio waves are bounced off the magnetic field, a computer records the results. Almost nothing else looks like the picture of MS lesions, and for most patients the MRI means a definite diagnosis.

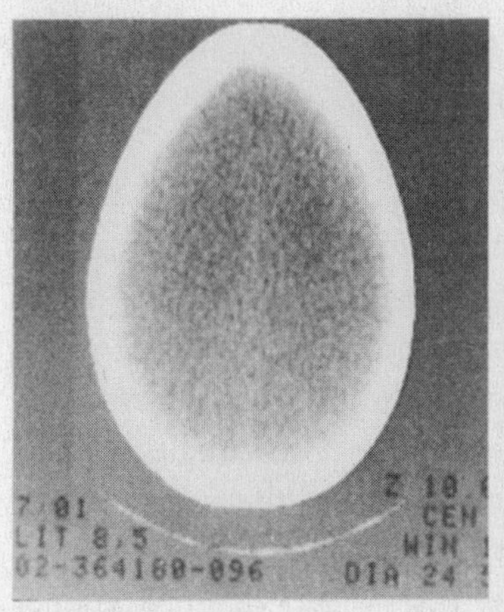

a

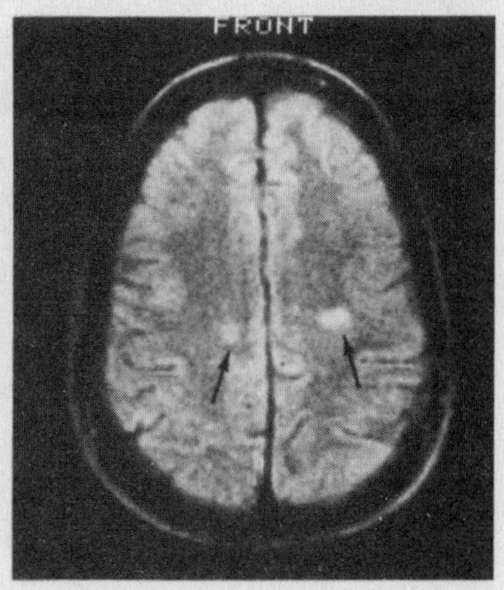

b

Cross sections of the CAT scan and the MRI: (a) front view, CAT scan; (b) front view, MRI; and (c) side view, MRI. Arrows indicate MS lesions.

(Photos courtesy Louis J. Rosner)

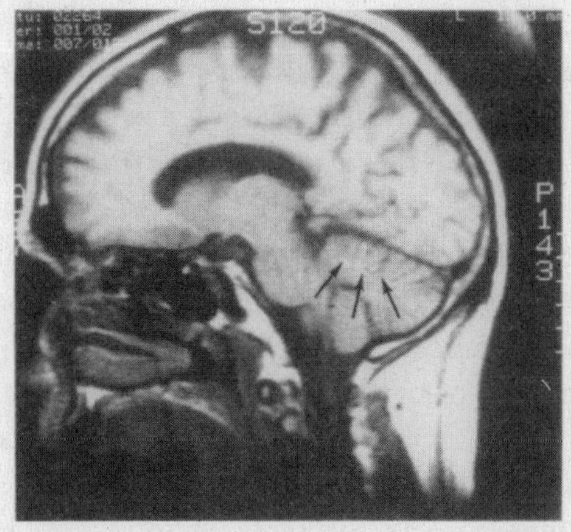

c

A DIAGNOSTIC CLASSIFICATION OF MULTIPLE SCLEROSIS

With the visualization of lesions made possible by the MRI, a doctor should be able to make an accurate diagnosis. But because lesions of other demyelinating diseases, such as SSPE, will show up on an MRI, the doctor must also rely on clinical judgment. Although it is a fantastic breakthrough, the MRI is in no way the single diagnostic test for MS. The doctor still must evaluate the results in the context of the patient's history and neurological examination.

Most doctors use three categories for MS diagnoses: definite MS, probable MS, and possible MS.

1. Definite MS: This diagnosis presents a clinical picture in which the patient has attacks with recovery and signs and symptoms that point to lesions in more than one location (optic nerve, brain stem, spinal cord, or cerebrum). All other reasonable possibilities are excluded, and one of three crucial lab tests, especially the MRI, shows typical MS findings.
2. Probable MS: In this diagnosis the clinical picture shows attacks with recovery, but the attacks may be all in the same spot; or there is evidence of more than one spot but no recovery or remission; or the lab tests are negative, which is not uncommon in an early case. Spinal fluid findings can be normal if tests are done when the disease is inactive. When the lesions are in the spinal cord only, they can be difficult to see, even with the MRI, and the MRI brain scan can also often be normal in the first three months of the disease.
3. Possible MS: This diagnosis is given when the lab tests are inconclusive but MS is still a possibility (along with others). The patient may have had only one attack,

symptoms in only one spot, or a slowly progressive illness without the more common course of attacks and remission.

Misdiagnosis of MS

The neurologist's office is often the court of last resort, where a patient winds up when all else fails. But there, too, misdiagnosis can and does happen. Despite the great advances in its diagnosis, MS is a disease with many variables. The misdiagnosis can either be a false negative, in which MS is missed, or a false positive, in which a patient is told that he or she has MS instead of another disease.

A false negative can occur when the patient has symptoms but no abnormal findings. Often a history of psychological disturbance can play a part. One woman, complaining of numbness in her hands and feet, stumped physicians for two months; she had no abnormal findings and she was a neurotic personality. Although she had MS, her problems were originally written off as psychological.

Other common misdiagnoses include the MS symptom of dizziness diagnosed as evidence of Ménière's syndrome, an inner ear ailment; the MS symptom of numbness or weakness in the limbs diagnosed as a pinched nerve or slipped disc in the neck or lower back; and the MS symptom of double vision diagnosed as resulting from stroke or drug abuse.

Thc false positive is not uncommon, either. In two studies of patients, conducted twenty years apart, between 9 and 12 percent of patients diagnosed with MS actually had other specific diseases. Another 5 percent of patients were mistakenly diagnosed as having MS, while the other disease they actually had remained unknown.

In many cases patients with small tumors were misdiagnosed as having MS. In one study tumors accounted for 95 percent of lesions misdiagnosed as MS. Doctors admit that even the MRI would not have helped in some of these cases. What can complicate matters even further is that steroid treatment, intended for MS patients, can often help patients with small tumors or inflammatory disease. When this occurs it can easily be misinterpreted as a typical MS remission.

Symptoms of many other diseases can mimic MS. Besides tumors, these include stroke, infection (notably viral encephalitis), mononucleosis, and neuritis. Neuritis can be due to an inflammation of the nerves, a pinched nerve, or compression of the nerve root by a disc. Disease arising from pressure on the spinal cord in the neck by a bulging disc mimics MS even more, since it comes on with slowly developing sensory or motor symptoms that can have periods of improvement. Sometimes there is a toxic cause of symptoms, which the patient conceals from the doctor: Alcoholism, for example, can cause loss of balance, double vision, or slurred speech.

Just as MS can be misdiagnosed as a psychological problem, a psychological problem can also be misdiagnosed as MS. Symptoms such as dizziness, fatigue, numbness, tingling, weakness, and loss of balance can be purely "hysterical." In fact, it is not uncommon to see a patient with MS and hysterical symptoms. A patient with a definite MS diagnosis might develop significant problems that are completely psychological and unrelated to the actual disease. A basic rule, however, is never to assume that a new complaint is another manifestation of MS. A new complaint could be psychological or due to another cause.

On what basis should a misdiagnosis be suspected? There are a few red flags to be aware of. They do not necessarily signal a misdiagnosis, but they suggest a need for medical reevaluation.

1. Although some cases with onset before age ten or after age fifty have been reported, this is so rare that an MS diagnosis is suspect. This is also true for onset prior to age forty of the rarer type of MS, which is without remission. Called "primary-progressive" MS, this is usually seen in patients with onset after age forty.
2. When the lesion is at the junction of the skull and cervical spine it can often appear as if there are two separate lesions, with the brain stem and spinal cord both affected. This can actually be a single lesion such as a tumor. Here the MRI is crucial in the diagnosis.
3. Hemianoptic field defects, in which half of the visual field (right or left) is impaired in both eyes, are so rare in MS that it is prudent to investigate other causes.
4. Geographical background that is inconsistent with the well-defined pattern of the world's MS population should make an MS diagnosis questionable. For example, if a patient grew up in the tropics or in a part of Asia where MS is extremely rare, other diseases, such as those caused by parasites, must be considered before MS.
5. Pain as a predominant symptom renders a diagnosis of MS suspect. Pain, as discussed in chapter 2, can be a symptom of MS. In fact, it is seen in up to 30 percent of patients at some point in the course of the disease. However, there are only a few kinds of pain associated with MS; others should be considered suspicious.
6. A so-called family history of MS should be cause for caution. Since there is such a low incidence of MS in families, there is a possibility that the entire family has been misdiagnosed and may actually suffer from another neurological disorder—a heredo-degenerative disease.

When the Diagnosis Is MS

For many, a positive (and accurate) MS diagnosis comes as a relief after weeks, months, often years of uncertainty. But for others, the diagnosis is a shock that hits hard. As diagnoses are made faster and faster with the increased use of the MRI, the impact can hit even harder. It is now possible to make a definite clinical diagnosis of MS within one week of onset. When should a doctor inform a patient of the diagnosis? If the diagnosis is definite MS, there is no question that the patient should be informed immediately. Sometimes the family is informed first and asks the doctor to keep the diagnosis a secret from the patient. Almost always, this is not a wise decision; every patient has the right to know.

When the diagnosis is probable or possible MS, the question becomes cloudier. With a probable diagnosis, most doctors feel the patient should be told after these questions are considered: How sure is the neurologist? How bad is the patient's case? Has the patient expressed the desire to know? Some patients don't want to know until the doctor is absolutely sure; they need to deal with the diagnosis in their own time.

A few years ago I was called to testify as an expert witness in a case brought against a neurologist who had told his patient everything about her disease but had never used the actual words *multiple sclerosis.* At the time she was actually classified as only a probable case, and he was reluctant to be more definite. Unfortunately, the patient left a job with solid medical benefits only to find herself a year later with a second MS attack and no insurance. Although a jury awarded her $100,000, no legal precedents were set and the issue will probably be debated for a long time.

With possible MS, which is basically just a suspicion, the

patient is usually not told unless he or she asks directly. This is touchy since the diagnosis often turns out to be something else.

The MRI is helping doctors zero in on more definite MS diagnoses than ever before. Oddly enough, there are some who regard this as a curse. One Los Angeles neurologist preferred the "good old days," when patients were "spared" the MS diagnosis for five or six prime years of their lives. We disagree wholeheartedly. An earlier, clear-cut diagnosis is much better. Since an MS diagnosis is not the end of the world, the sooner one hears it, the sooner one can learn to cope with it and get on with life accordingly. For example, a woman might choose to have a baby sooner, while she knows her MS is more likely to remain in a mild stage and she is better equipped to deal with a toddler. Another person might choose not to have children at all; priorities might now be to return to graduate or law school. An MS diagnosis will no doubt change a person's life, and no one is saying it's easy to deal with. But it's foolish to think anyone would be better off not knowing.

Often the people who cope best with an MS diagnosis are those who have doctors who can cope with it. Even today, many doctors who are uncomfortable with the diagnosis will use vague or obscure euphemisms such as "inflammation of the nervous system," "a disease of myelin," or "a neurological problem that may come and go." This can keep patients in limbo. In general, it is best that the patient be told, without hesitation, "Your diagnosis is multiple sclerosis. Let me explain what that means."

Because the best-informed patient is the one who will fare best, no one should be afraid to go to another neurologist for a second opinion. And no one should be too embarrassed to ask the first doctor to forward test results and records. A good neurologist will understand and even encourage this. Those who don't know of any other neurologist can ask their family physicians to recommend one or call their local branch of the American Medical Association or National Multiple Sclerosis Society and ask for the names of a few board-certified neurologists. Medical schools or teaching hospitals can be of help, too.

4

The Course

"What's going to happen to me?"

That's the most natural question asked by the person diagnosed with MS. Unfortunately, the course of MS is unpredictable at best. At one extreme there are "silent" cases in which no neurological symptoms are ever seen, yet MS lesions are found through testing or at autopsy. At the other extreme are those who get progressively worse right from the start, without any recovery. In between are the majority of MS patients, who have a number of attacks with recovery.

Like other diseases, MS has mild forms and more serious forms. Think of arthritis, for example. Some people will only get a sore elbow when it rains, while others suffer far more debilitating effects. MS actually has four known courses—benign, relapsing-remitting, secondary-progressive, and primary-progressive.

The benign course is characterized by a sudden onset. The patient will report only one or two mild attacks with complete or nearly complete remission. There will be no disability involved.

The relapsing-remitting course also has a sudden onset.

The patient has relapses with remissions and suffers no permanent damage. These patients experience no restrictions in their daily activities and tend to remain gainfully employed. There are often long periods of remission.

The secondary-progressive course starts out with attacks with full remissions, but five or more years after onset it will turn progressive.

The primary-progressive course involves a slow worsening without remission. The onset is much slower. In some patients the permanent damage can be severely disabling; in others, it is not.

One of the most difficult issues for people with MS to face is not knowing which course their MS will take. Only after following a patient for five or six years will a neurologist be able to make an educated prediction. The unpredictability of MS is one of its most frustrating factors; patients and their families are, of course, anxious to make career, family, and financial plans. Though it may be easier to assess the course of an individual's disease after five years, most newly diagnosed patients want answers sooner.

Although there are no crystal balls, it does help to examine the available statistics along with accepted indicators of a good prognosis. Basically, the odds are in the patient's favor. At least 20 percent of people with MS will have a benign course. About 20 to 30 percent will have a relapsing-remitting course. Approximately 40 percent of people with MS will have a relapsing-remitting course that becomes progressive. Of this group, half will have only slight permanent damage, such as mild weakness in one leg. The other half will progress over many years to a more serious disability. Only 10 to 20 percent, mostly older onset patients, will have primary-progressive course. And only a small percentage of those will become severely disabled, unable to care for themselves.

Seventy-five percent of all MS patients will remain ambulatory, never needing a wheelchair. MS is almost never a cause of death. When the disease does shorten the life span, it is usually because of secondary infections, which can usually be prevented by proper medical care. Since the mid-1950s, the life span of people with MS has increased by ten years. Those with MS can now expect to live out at least 90 percent of a normal life span.

Onset as a Clue to Prognosis

Although most doctors are reluctant to suggest a prognosis before five years, researchers have analyzed some early indicators. Age of onset, for instance, plays a strong role in a person's prognosis. When the first symptoms appear in the twenties and thirties, the person has a better chance of getting a mild form of MS. On the other hand, onset in the teens or forties puts the person at a higher risk of ultimately entering a progressive stage.

In one of the best studies other indicators were analyzed. Using the patient records of the University of Washington MS Clinic, along with two hundred books and articles and the opinions of directors of thirty MS clinics throughout the country, researchers identified characteristics that point to a good prognosis. They include onset on or before age thirty-five (we believe it is age forty), one symptom at onset, one symptom during the first year, sudden appearance of symptoms, initial remission within one month, little or no residual deficit after each exacerbation, absence of ataxia and the Babinski sign at the initial examination, optic neuritis or other sensory signs as the sole presenting symptom, brief duration of the most recent exacerbation, current ambulatory ability, minimal ataxia (loss of balance), and minimal pyramidal signs (abnormal reflexes) five years after onset.

Coordination trouble and motor weakness were shown to be stronger indicators of eventual disability.

Frequency and Duration of Attack

In most cases the first attack of MS clears completely within four to six weeks, often leaving no trace of abnormality on neurological examination. Many years can lapse between the first and second attack. In a French study of 114 remitting patients, the periods between the first and second attacks were the following: 20 relapsed within the first six months, 27 within six to twelve months, 20 within one to two years, 25 within two to five years, 13 within five to ten years, and 9 after ten years. The longest time period recorded in this study between the first and second attack was seventeen years.

The frequency of attacks is related to the duration of the disease. In the early stages bouts can occur once, twice, even three times a year. In the middle stages they will decrease to an average of one attack every few years. The prognosis for recovery or improvement from an attack seems to be related to the duration of the bout.

Spontaneous Cure

Some patients will have several severe attacks in the first five years, casting an ominous shadow over the future. But then the disease will stop spontaneously, there will be no more attacks, and the patient will return to normal or near normal. It's as if the disease just burned itself out.

Dramatic recoveries have occurred in patients with seemingly severe damage. It is these "miracles" that lead to claims for various treatments from quack cures to faith healing.

One of the most incredible turnarounds I personally observed was in a patient who at age thirty-eight had a devastating attack. She went into a convulsion and was left in a state of stupor—unable to talk, walk, or use her arms or legs at all. She was blind, had severely slurred speech, and could not swallow or even stay awake. Unable to care for herself at home, she was hospitalized. Since she did not respond to standard treatment, her prognosis was very gloomy. In fact, it appeared that she would never recover. Incredibly, however, she made a slow improvement in the hospital and eventually returned completely to normal. Her recovery was not due to treatment but apparently due to some body defense system. And for the next twelve years, her MS continued on a mild relapsing-remitting course.

What Is It Really Like as MS Takes Its Course over the Years?

Charts and statistics can provide some information, but the only way to get a real understanding of what the person with MS typically faces is to look at real case studies.

In private practice, I often discharged patients with very mild or benign cases after reasonable periods of remission. But I also followed many private patients, for as long as thirty years, with the classic challenges of MS. The first 7 patients we review here illustrate the natural course of the disease before 1993 when new medications became available on the market which can actually modify the disease and change the course of MS in many people. Of my 60 regular patients I treated before 1993, more than half were relapsing-remitting; 25 percent were secondary-progressive; the rest were primary-progressive. We've selected these case studies because they are realistic, some even gritty. They are the best examples of people who have lived with the many twists and turns of MS.

Later, after we examine these 7 patients who didn't have the benefits of the newest pharmaceutical treatments early in their course, we'll look at some who have.

Relapsing-Remitting Course

C. M., female, age forty-seven in 1990, had a relapsing-remitting course of attacks with remissions for twenty-five years. Her onset was in March 1966 at age twenty-three when she experienced numbness and tingling in the entire left leg. It cleared in six weeks.

May 1968—The second attack started with blurred vision in her right eye, with a total loss of vision over five days. With cortisone treatment it improved but never completely returned to normal.

December 1969—Then four months pregnant, C. M. had some vision loss in her left eye. With cortisone it improved within two weeks and returned to normal by one month.

August 1972—C. M. experienced numbness in the left leg to the waist, which cleared within two weeks.

March 1974—Numbness now occurred in the right leg and lower trunk, with complete recovery within two weeks.

June 1975—C. M. reported double vision with complete recovery within nine days.

July 1977—A burning sensation accompanied numbness up the right leg to the lower trunk. Recovery was in four weeks.

December 1977—The numbness in the right leg returned, continuing up the trunk to the shoulder. C. M. also felt weakness in her left arm. The attack lasted two months before she returned to normal.

August 1978—After spraining her left knee in an

accident in which she slipped and fell, C. M. had a new attack in which she experienced weakness in her left leg for one year and then completely recovered.

January 1990—After twelve years in remission, which included a remarriage, gall bladder surgery, colds, a fungus infection, and dental work, C. M. had a new attack, experiencing tingling in the right foot, numbness, and weakness in the right leg, which spread to the rib cage. With prednisone, C. M. returned to normal within three weeks.

June 1990—Periodontal surgery with no attack.

C. M. continued to work as a marriage and family counselor, remaining in remission with just a slight visual loss, an old residual symptom of the right eye. This case illustrates one typical pattern: a stormy course the first few years, then a benign course with rare attacks and no permanent damage.

B. B., female, by age thirty-nine had a relapsing-remitting course for twenty-six years. Her onset was in 1964 at age thirteen, although it was not diagnosed at the time. She experienced numbness in the hands and legs and tingling down the back on bending the head to the chest. Within two weeks, she returned to normal.

At some time in 1965, she went blind in the right eye for five minutes, but no connection was made to her earlier symptom.

October 1971—After a bout with viral hepatitis that lasted one month, she developed dizziness, loss of balance, and double vision. After five days she returned to normal.

February 1972—B. B. tripped on the stairs and sprained her left ankle. Two days later her left foot was numb. The numbness then climbed to the but-

tocks, then rose to the same level on the right side. By the tenth day of the attack, the numbness had moved to the waist. At this point she was hospitalized and given a myelogram, which was normal. The numbness improved, and she returned to normal.

June 1972—The day after experiencing flu symptoms and going through an emotional crisis over a boyfriend, she had a new attack of tingling in the legs, along with numbness from the head down the arms and legs. Her right hand was clumsy. Her right leg was weak and stiff, and she experienced a girdle sensation around the trunk. She also felt a tight band around her right knee and a numbness in the right side of her face and head. At that point the diagnosis of MS was made, and she was treated with cortisone. She recovered in two and a half months.

January 1973—A flare-up of herpes virus in her mouth (a cold sore) precipitated another attack of numbness on the left side from the breast down, which spread to the right side from the breast down. She also had weakness of the legs with numbness, and stiffness and clumsiness of the hands. It lasted two months and she returned to normal.

August 1976—After a mild stomach ailment, she had a one-month attack of numbness from the bust to the waistline.

February 1977—B. B. experienced weakness in the left arm and leg lasting eighteen days before she returned to normal.

July 1977—For three weeks she had numbness in the left face and hand, which returned to normal.

September 1977—A new attack resulted in numbness and weakness in the left leg for one week before she returned to normal.

June 1978—Weakness in the left leg lasted for five days before she returned to normal.

September 1978—B. B. got married.

October 1978—She experienced numbness and weakness in the right leg for five days.

July 1979—She had weakness in the left arm and leg with tingling down the back on bending the head forward. The attack lasted six weeks, then she returned to normal.

February 1980—For one month she had numbness in the left arm and leg, along with a decrease in vision in the right eye. She returned to normal.

September 1981—Numbness in the right leg crept up the trunk to the armpit. This was accompanied by weakness in the right leg, unsteady walk, and hypersensitivity in the left arm. After two months she returned to normal.

October 1983—For a period of two months, she experienced numbness in the left leg and trunk to the shoulder blade, then returned to normal.

March 1984—Tingling and tightness on the left side of the trunk at the waist lasted for five weeks, then cleared completely.

June 1984—Weakness in the left leg lasted four days, then cleared completely.

August 1984—Numbness in the left trunk and leg lasted two days, then cleared completely.

November 1984—A tight girdle sensation around the trunk lasted for two days and cleared completely.

April 1985—She felt a burning sensation in the right leg, a heaviness in the left leg, and double vision. The symptoms disappeared in one month.

February 1986—She experienced numbness in the right hand, which spread to the right side, and then to the left hand and leg. She returned to normal in a little over a month.

June 1986—After exercise classes her right leg would become tired and numb. This stopped when she quit the classes.

August 1986—B. B. intermittently felt numbness in the left foot and leg and heaviness of the leg. Late in the day, or when she was on her feet too much, she would also feel burning or a "freezing" sensation on the soles of the feet. This remitted completely in two months.

October 1987—Weakness in limbs and numbness from the waist down, along with urinary incontinence, appeared with cold symptoms and a cold sore on the lip. With cortisone treatment, B. B. recovered within one month.

Febraury 1988—Weakness and tingling in the legs, along with an unsteady balance, followed a sore throat and another cold sore. B. B. recovered within a month without cortisone.

May 1988—Two brief episodes of complete numbness and inability to walk lasting only a few seconds.

September 1988—Weakness in the right hand and foot and numbness on the left side from the waist down. B. B. was responding well to prednisone when the next attack occurred.

November 1988—Numbness in the left arm and leg lasted for two weeks and B.B. recovered without treatment.

December 1988—Numbness and heaviness in the left arm and leg, tight girdle sensation around the trunk, and balance trouble was treated with cortisone for two and a half weeks. B. B. recovered fully in three and a half weeks.

> *April 1990—B. B. experienced numbness and dragging of the left leg and recovered in three months without treatment.*
>
> *September 1990—Numbness and weakness in the right arm and leg. B. B. recovered in one week without treatment.*
>
> *October 1990—Blisters on the lip and sinus trouble were followed by hypersensitivity to touch and a "frozen" feeling in the right hand, along with numbness and tightness in the left hand and weakness in both legs. Recovery was within three months with prednisone treatment and Tegretol for the pain.*

In twenty-seven years she had thirty-two attacks, and each time she returned completely to normal. Each year is different, some good, some challenging. She remains happily married.

Secondary-Progressive Course

> *K. L., female, age forty-four in 1990, had the onset of MS in 1963 at age sixteen. At the time she experienced numbness and tingling in her feet, which spread to the waist. It peaked in a week and stayed at the peak for one month. The symptoms disappeared the following month, and no diagnosis was made.*
>
> *July 1964—She had pain in the right eye upon movement, along with loss of central vision. Her eye doctor diagnosed her case as optic neuritis. She recovered completely in four weeks.*
>
> *December 1966—She lost vision in her left eye and returned to normal within one month. At the time she was told her diagnosis was "probable" MS, while reinforcing that it was not a bad case. She went*

to college, and unfortunately the doctor at the student health service told her she'd wind up in a wheelchair.

July 1967—She started a new summer job in sales, which involved standing on her feet for long periods of time. After three weeks on the job, she felt numbness in her left leg to the waist, along with heaviness in the same leg. With cortisone treatment she was well within two and a half weeks.

October 1967—At college she had numbness in the right face, arm, leg, and trunk. With cortisone treatment she returned to normal in five weeks.

December 1967—She felt numbness from the waist down, which lasted three months.

August 1968—After starting work as a student teacher, she was married.

April 1970—After suffering a common bladder infection that was not related to MS or any neurological cause, she had an attack that caused numbness in the left leg and trunk up to the waist. She described a strange sensation of having "super-thick skin like an elephant." After six weeks she completely recovered.

July 1971—K. L. had her first baby, with no neurological episodes.

March 1972—She experienced numbness in the left hand and right leg and trunk up to the waist. She also had tingling in the arms and legs upon bending the head. This disappeared in one month.

April 1972—As soon as she recovered from the last attack, she felt numbness again in both legs up to the waist. She also had stiffness in the legs and a clumsy gait that lasted two months, and then she recovered.

January 1973—Her vision wavered on looking from side to side. She felt weakness and had jerky eye movements. With cortisone she recovered within four weeks.

February 1973—Once again she experienced an attack of numbness, this time lasting five months and affecting her right arm, both legs, and lower trunk. By July she returned to normal.

September 1973—A short attack of numbness from the legs up to the waist lasted four days before clearing completely.

March 1976—K. L. had a second baby with no neurological episodes.

July 1977—Both legs became numb as did the left side of the face. Her balance was off, and she developed double vision. With cortisone all symptoms cleared in two weeks.

October 1977—She felt weakness in the right hand and leg. With cortisone she recovered in one month.

December 1977—For two weeks she experienced a weak and clumsy hand. Then she returned to normal.

January 1978—For one week she had double, blurred vision and a cross-eyed appearance. She returned to normal.

November 1979—She had another attack of numbness in the legs, this time with dizziness, unsteady balance, and trouble focusing her eyes. With cortisone treatment this cleared in six weeks.

June 1980—She developed a limp in her right leg along with balance trouble. Her right arm was weak and stiff. Her eyes felt weak upon looking to the left. With cortisone treatment all symptoms cleared in one month.

July 1985—She experienced weakness in the right foot and up the whole leg and numbness in both legs to the waist. With cortisone treatment the numbness cleared completely after six weeks, but the right leg remained slightly weak from then on.

January 1986—While running down an incline on a slippery surface, she slipped and fell. The trauma brought on a new attack. She felt dizzy, her eyes became weak, and she had trouble focusing when looking to each side. With cortisone treatment she returned to normal within ten days except for the old mild leg weakness.

June 1986—After doing a lot of walking, her right leg got weaker, causing her to fall two times in one week. After treatment with cortisone, the leg got better but only came back to the previous status. Because the leg did not come back to normal and had remained weak for one year, her case could no longer be classified as relapsing-remitting. It was now secondary-progressive.

June 1986—Later that month her left leg collapsed, and she described it as feeling like jelly at the ankle. She developed incoordination of both legs and had an unsteady balance. The left leg recovered by the next day, and, with cortisone, the right leg improved again.

October 1986—The right leg got weaker again, but improved with a retrial of cortisone.

January 1987—K. L. returned to school to work on her master's degree in psychology.

April 1978—For the first time, during a group therapy session, she revealed her MS diagnosis to others.

October 1987—K. L. had a modified left mastectomy for breast cancer with no change in her MS symptoms.

June 1988—Stiffness and weakness in the right leg was treated with cortisone, but did not return to normal. Cortisone was stopped after two months. Her husband filed for divorce.

October 1990—Residual right leg weakness remains unchanged since 1988.

K. L. had an episodic course for more than twenty-two years before becoming progressive. She's had two reconstructive breast surgeries without MS activity. In 1989 she began working at a psychotherapy clinic. When outside the house, she uses a cane for support. Her case illustrates the mild nature of some residual MS damage after a long episodic stage.

L.S., a seventy-four-year-old male dentist, may have had his first MS attack in 1944, at age twenty-eight. At the time he fractured his left leg in an auto accident and soon after experienced numbness in that leg from the knee down. His next episode wasn't for twenty years.

1964—At age forty-eight he found himself dragging his left leg, which recovered on its own after one week.

August 1966—He experienced motion sickness, balance difficulty, and ringing in the ear. It was (mis)diagnosed as Ménière's disease and cleared in one week.

December 1966—He felt numbness in the left arm. He returned to normal after four days.

April 1967—He had pain in the right eye upon movement, which lasted one week. He also had a blind spot for one morning. The diagnosis was optic neuritis, and he was treated with cortisone. The central vision loss in the right eye slowly improved but never returned to normal.

July 1967—L. S. had numbness in the left side of the tongue and mouth and experienced loss of taste. One month later he had trouble focusing. This was followed by weakness on the left side of his face, ringing in the left ear, and unsteady walk. At this time the MS diagnosis was made. After treatment with cortisone, he returned to normal in three months.

February 1968—This attack marked the end of the relapsing-remitting course. It began with numbness in the left arm and weakness in the left hand and leg. One week later he lost vision in the right eye. With cortisone the right eye recovered in two weeks. But the weakness in the left hand and leg never returned to normal. He has had a permanent weakenss ever since.

August 1970—After physical exhaustion the weakness in the left leg increased, and he developed tingling in the right leg along with loss of balance. He improved but was left with more weakness in the left leg than before.

1971—During the year the left leg got slowly weaker. There was a little improvement with cortisone treatment, but the weakness was worse than the year before.

During 1972, 1973, and 1974, the weak left leg remained the same. In 1975, while he was under emotional strain, his left leg slowly worsened.

March 1983—The right leg became slightly weak.

August 1984—He fell coming out of a swimming pool. The left leg became weaker than ever.

January 1986—He experienced paresthesias of the left leg, the feeling of "water" on the skin. He had trouble focusing his eyes and had numbness of the left arm and left leg. With cortisone treatment he recovered from the new symptoms in six weeks.

June 1986—New weakness appeared in the right hand and right leg, along with sharp shooting pains in the left lower jaw to the ear. Without medication he recovered from the new symptoms in one week.

July 1986—L. S. began to use a crutch to walk. Face pains were relieved with Dilantin.

October 1986—He began to experience dizzy spells from changing positions too quickly; his left arm and leg became weaker.

January 1988—He began to fall due to loss of balance.

March 1988—Prostate surgery caused temporary postoperative urinary incontinence. The left leg got weaker and dragged more.

July 1988—The strength in the left hand and leg improved.

April 1989—His left arm and leg became weaker after surgery on the left shoulder to repair an injury.

January 1990—The left arm and leg improved.

April 1990—L. S. retired from dentistry after forty-four years.

L. S. had a relapsing-remitting course for the first four years of his illness. If the 1944 numbness following the car accident is included, the relapsing-remitting course lasted twenty-four years. Since 1976 the weakness in the legs and hand has fluctuated and is directly related to how much he is overworked, overtired, and overexerted. Today he has severe weakness in the left leg and uses a knee brace. He also has mild weakness in the left hand. He walks with a crutch and still works part-time treating jaw-joint disorders. This case illustrates what may happen with older age of onset: a short-duration relapsing-remitting stage and more severe permanent damage.

S.M., male, age forty-eight in 1990, had his first episode of MS in 1978 at age thirty-six. He experienced dizziness and tingling in the left neck and shoulder, which lasted two weeks.

January 1980—Two weeks after a short bout with the flu, he had his second MS attack. He felt tingling in his left hand and up the arm followed by numbness and hypersensitivity in the left hand and arm and up the left side to the neck for seven days. After a myelogram was normal, the diagnosis of MS was made. He was treated with cortisone, showed improvement, and returned to normal in three months except for hypersensitivity of the hands.

August 1980—He developed weakness of the left leg, which slowly worsened and would vary in intensity depending on use. If he walked too much, it became worse; if he rested, it got better. After three months the leg returned to normal, and he went on a trip to the Far East, visiting Hong Kong, Singapore, and Bali. After three weeks the leg became weak again, although only slightly.

February 1984—A new attack was marked by double vision, which cleared in one month. The left leg continued to be very slightly weak.

April 1984—The left hand became weak and clumsy and returned to normal by December.

April 1985—The weakness in the left leg worsened, and the left hand became weak again. Cortisone did not improve the condition, and throughout 1985 the left hand and leg stayed weak.

October 1985—The right leg became weak for the first time.

November 1985—He went into an experimental treatment program, and after receiving immunosup-

pressant drugs, he got temporarily better. The hand returned to normal and the left leg was stronger.

January 1986—After another bout with the flu, his left hand and leg got weaker again.

May 1986—A new attack further weakened the left leg and hand. He also experienced splotchy vision. Cortisone was tried in addition to immunosuppressant drugs but did not help.

July 1986—Weakness appeared on the right side in the leg and hand.

August 1987—S. M. had increased weakness in all four limbs, which improved slightly after treatment with cortisone for four months.

January 1988—Flu did not worsen symptoms.

July 1988—Leg weakness worsened. Treatment with ACTH was not helpful. After six weeks, weakness worsened more. He now needed support to walk.

August 1988—After weakness in hands and legs worsened, he began treatment with chlorambucil, which continued monthly until 1989. S. M. improved for six months, then slowly worsened again.

September 1989—Intravenous cortisone was not helpful.

August 1990—Gold injections were tried and stopped after one month.

November 1990—S. M. began using a wheelchair because of increased leg weakness.

Today S. M. still runs his own real estate company and continues to work full time. His weakness is now severe. This case illustrates a typical story for this type of MS in which the spinal cord is the main site of involvement and weakness of the legs is the main symptom. The relapsing-remitting stage is usually short. He has tried many experimental treatments, but to no avail.

Primary-Progressive Course

A. H., female, age fifty-six in 1990, had her onset in April 1972 at age thirty-eight, with an episode of visual loss that was diagnosed as inflammation and treated with cortisone. The vision came back, but not completely.

During 1976—After playing tennis, she noticed her right leg would become fatigued and begin to drag. Gradually the leg got worse, and it took less exertion to bring on the fatigue.

Winter 1977—She experienced a cold feeling in the right leg from the knee down.

1978—After continued weakness in the right hip and ankle, the first neurological evaluation was conducted in the hospital. The tests included X-ray, myelogram, spinal fluid studies, and visual evoked response tests. All were normal, and a diagnosis was not made in spite of the thoroughness.

1979—A CAT scan was performed because she now had weakness in the right hand—a symptom suggesting a spot in the brain, not the spinal cord. The results were normal.

November 1980—A. H. had blurred vision in the right eye and her visual evoked response tests were abnormal. At this time an MS diagnosis was made on the basis of two separate spots of involvement. The right vision came back almost to normal, but in hot weather or when she was tired, the right eye would blur. It also would be better with rest or worse later in the day.

1981 on—She had slow worsening, with weakness of the right hand and right leg, but no new acute attacks.

At the present, A. H. has moderate weakness in the right hand and leg. She tires easily, and now walks with a cane or other support.

A. H. is married, with three grown children. She needs some help with the housework. Her story illustrates the mild character of some primary-progressive cases in which after eighteen years of symptoms, there is only a moderate disability. Interestingly, some limitations in A. H.'s life are due to emotional, not physical, problems.

E. L., male, sixty-six in 1990, had MS onset late in life. In March 1975, at age fifty, he had an accident in which he fell off a box onto his back. He experienced low back pain and weakness of the legs. With bed rest he improved and was able to walk, but with a limp in his right leg.

August 1977—His right leg was worse, dragging when he walked; he had to lift the leg with his hand to move it. Two myelograms did not reveal a diagnosis.

August 1978—His right hand became weak and stayed weak. With cortisone he showed improvement in the hand, but not in the right leg.

November 1978—The left hand and leg became slightly weak. Cortisone for three weeks did not help.

April 1979—Spinal tap findings were positive for MS.

July 1982—The weakness in the left leg became a little worse, and he began to use a cane and a right leg brace.

March 1983—The right leg was even weaker.

February 1984—The right leg worsened again.

May 1984—He began to use a walker.

January 1985—The left leg was weaker.

May 1986—The weakness in hands and legs was more severe on the right side. He began to use a wheelchair.

August 1986—The left leg got better, and E. L. was able to return to use of a walker while inside.

May 1988—Arm strength improved.

August 1988—His legs weakened.

March 1989—His leg weakness worsened.

June 1989—E. L.'s condition was better, but weakness persisted.

August 1990—He improved, but was still weak in all four limbs.

E. L.'s case is typical of primary-progressive MS, which begins late in life. Although this form of MS represents 10 to 20 percent of all cases, it is the most challenging since disability is insidious and without remission. But this case shows that even primary-progressive MS can take a turn for the better after years of slow worsening. E. L. lives independently. His wife works, he takes care of the house.

The New Frontier

The next two cases illustrate the influence of the new disease-modifying agents in changing the course of MS. These new cutting-edge treatments, often have dramatic results and will be discussed in greater depth in chapters 6 and 11. But first some background.

In 1993, the first drug was released that could stop relapses and prevent the change from relapsing MS to progressive MS. This was interferon beta-1B (Betaseron). Two years later, interferon beta-1A (Avonex) became available. And in 1996, the drug glatiramer (Copaxone) was added to the list. The outlook for early cases of MS was immensely improved. If put on one of these medications right away, a newly diagnosed patient stood a good chance of having infrequent or no relapses and never going into the progressive stage of the disease. Patients who have had relapsing-remitting MS for some time and are worsening could benefit greatly. Also MRI lesions of MS often were reduced or disappeared. Again, after this chapter we will discuss how these innovations came about, why the drugs are supposed to work, whether or not they have lived up to their promise, and what is the downside of taking them.

> *R. R., female, now fifty-three, had the onset of MS in June 1978 at the age of twenty-five. Initial symptoms were blurred vision, double vision, trouble focusing, headache, lightheadedness, dizziness, unsteadiness, lack of coordination, and dropping things. This episode lasted seven to nine days. On examination she had nystagmus of the eyes, which recovered in two months.*
>
> *May 1982—Headache, tingling spreading up the right leg, tense feeling in the right hand and arm, and dizziness were symptoms of the second attack. Two days later she had numbness of the trunk up to the right breast, and right leg weakness. Improvement began two days later.*
>
> *June 1982—She had numbness, tingling, and weakness in the left hand and leg, which cleared in four weeks.*
>
> *October 1982—She had numbness and tingling in the left face and hand for two weeks.*

May 1983—Pain in the left eye on movement and cloudiness of vision in this eye with finding of a central blind spot (scotoma) led to a diagnosis of optic neuritis and treatment with prednisone. She recovered in eight days.

July 1983—Another episode of left optic neuritis occurred and was treated with prednisone; she recovered in six days.

September 1983—She had two days of tingling in the left face and fingers.

January 1984—She developed dizziness, spinning feeling, lightheadedness, pain in the arms and legs, and tingling in the left fingers lasting five days.

March 1984—R. R. gave birth to her first baby.

August 1984—She had another episode of left optic neuritis, was treated with prednisone, and recovered in four days.

November 1984—She had pain in the left eye and was again given prednisone and recovered in five days.

February 1985—She had heaviness of the legs and a tight band across the chest for two days.

June 1985—Tingling in the right fingers and toes was treated with niacin.

April 1987—R. R. developed left-sided numbness and weakness, accompanying infections and dizziness. The symptoms went away in a few days.

October 1988—R. R. was pregnant for the second time. She had tingling and pains in the legs with positive Lhermitte's sign for a short time.

June 1989—Her second baby was born.

June 1990—Optic neuritis in the right eye was treated with prednisone for two weeks and she recovered in eighteen days.

April 1991—R. R. had another episode of right optic neuritis, and was treated with prednisone with recovery in twelve days.

April 1992—While in Mexico, R. R. had an episode of right eye pain and right arm and leg weakness. It was hot and humid and there was no air conditioning.

January 1993—She had hypersensitivity, pain, and heaviness in both arms for one week.

January 1994—R. R. was started on Betaseron.

January 1995—She had a two-day episode of stiffness in her legs.

April 1995—She had heaviness, fatigue, pain, and hypersensitivity in her legs for a short time.

February 1996—She had fatigue and pain in her legs.

September 1996—After two years, eight months, use of Betaseron was stopped and Avonex was started because of its convenient once-a-week use instead of every other day.

August 1997—R. R. had a relapse with slurred speech and tingling in her legs. She took steroids (Medrol) for six days. The symptoms remitted and she was normal again except for slurred speech when tired. MRI of the head and spine showed active lesions all over.

January 1998—She had fatigue and slurred speech, was treated with Cylert and then amantadine.

May 1998—Two days after an Avonex injection she developed fatigue, sleepiness, and slurred speech. Avonex was stopped because of continued relapses and worsening of MRI. Relapse persisted with new symptoms of numbness of the feet and lower legs. She took Medrol for six days and symptoms gradually went away.

July 1998—R. R. started Copaxone.

September 1998—She relapsed with pain, tingling, and weakness in the legs, then numbness of the whole right side. She took Medrol for six days, then prednisone for ten days. This relapse lasted fifty-two days during which time she needed support when walking because of leg weakness.

April 1999—She had an episode of slurred speech and numbness of the right fingers.

August 1999—She had an episode of slurred speech and trouble with word-finding problems.

April 2000—She had an episode of slurred speech and fatigue, treated with bed rest.

May 2001—She had an exacerbation with fatigue, leg pains, blurred vision, aching all over, and heaviness of the legs. She took prednisone and recovered.

August 2001—She had another episode of slurred speech, fatigue, and depression, and was treated with two days of bed rest.

December 2001—While doing yoga, her legs became shaky and painful. The next day she had heaviness of the legs, slurred speech, and depression, and could hardly move. After a course of oral steroids she recovered.

May 2002—She had a relapse with heaviness of the legs, fatigue, and depression treated with steroids.

July 2002—R. R. stopped Copaxone because of six attacks in four years, four of them were severe enough to require steroids. Betaseron was begun again.

August 2002—She had a new attack after five weeks on Betaseron with weak stiff legs for which she took Medrol for six days.

February 2003—She had right eye pain and poor vision which resolved in two days without treatment.

September 2002—She had depression, fatigue, and slurred speech, which were treated with bed rest for two days.

June 2003—She had another relapse requiring steroids.

September 2003—She had numbness in the arms and legs and a tight band around the chest that cleared after steroid treatment.

February 2004—She took prednisone for heaviness and weakness of the legs, and made a good recovery.

July 2004—She had headache, fatigue, and slurred speech, which were treated with two days of bed rest.

November 2004—She had tiredness, slurred speech and left leg weakness which resolved after steroid treatment.

December 2004—She took steroids again for leg weakness.

September 2005—She had an episode of slurred speech and slight right facial droop, requiring no treatment.

November 2005—She had "spasms" all over her body, was treated with IV steroids, and recovered.

Early 2006—Occasional episodes of slurred speech and fatigue were relieved by bed rest for two days.

October 2006—One week after a flu shot and during a period of great stress, she had an episode of right optic neuritis, was treated with prednisone, and recovered in three days.

R. R. has had relapsing-remitting MS for twenty-eight years. In the first fifteen years before the advent of the disease-modifying agents she had nineteen attacks. In the thirteen years since using these medications she has had nineteen attacks. This may not appear to be the great achievement it actually is. She has fully recovered every time. She has no permanent damage and no disability, only occasional slurred speech when fatigued. She continues to take care of her home, husband, children, and dog. She does the down dogs and sun salutations of yoga as well as ever. And she is a renowned expert in fund raising. And most significant, she has never entered the secondary-progressive phase that was the likely, almost expected course of her MS.

> *W.R., a forty-nine-year-old female costume designer and cat lover, had the onset of MS in September 1997 at the age of forty. Initial symptoms were severe vertigo, ringing in the ears, tingling and funny feelings in the left leg, and urinary urgency. An MRI of the brain was positive. A spinal tap was negative. MS was diagnosed, and she was started on Copaxone within a month.*
>
> *September 1999—She had an episode of right eye blurring and headache, which may have been a migraine attack.*
>
> *October 1999—She had a bad migraine attack. Then she developed left face weakness and couldn't lift her left eyebrow; she had slowness of the left hand, slurred speech, and hoarse voice. These symptoms resolved after three to four weeks.*
>
> *June 2000—She had occasional left leg heaviness and soreness, going away with movement, and some blurring of vision in the right eye.*
>
> *December 2000—She had an episode of severe vertigo that resolved quickly, then a mild headache for two days. This was followed by transient numbness in her left fingers and left leg and hypersensitivity*

around the waist and left leg that went away after two months. There was also urinary urgency and one episode of urinary incontinence.

July 2001—Another flare-up occurred characterized by numbness of the left fingers and foot, a "smudge" in the outer right half of vision, a color disturbance in the right eye, and pain on eye movement. She recovered without treatment.

January 2002—She had migraines at the time of menstrual periods and visual symptoms when exercising at the gym.

July 2002—Migraines increased in intensity and frequency. There was an episode of iritis but no MS symptoms.

January 2003—Migraines increased at the time of her periods. MS symptoms consisted of "splotchy" vision when overheated and urinary urgency.

July 2003—She had headaches with menstrual periods. Her left leg felt heavy for a few hours.

August 2004—She had frequent migraines.

January 2005—For one week she had blurred vision and a scotoma in the right lower quadrant with light sensitivity. There were three migraine attacks, a little stiffness of the neck, and some incoordination of the hands. These symptoms were treated with steroids and she recovered.

February 2005—An MRI showed multiple lesions and enhancement. She was given steroids again for three days.

January 2006—She had an episode of iritis treated with prednisone eye drops. A tight band feeling around the abdomen occurred, lasting a few weeks.

February 2006—She had balance trouble and slurred speech, and her left eye felt weak. She went to an emergency room, got one dose of IV steroids, then took Medrol for six days. The symptoms resolved except for stiffness and weakness in the left leg which was not detectable on examination.

May 2006—She was back to normal except for a tight band feeling at the left waist, one episode of slurred speech, urinary urgency, and fecal urgency.

September 2006—She had a bad cold with dizziness, weakness, and nausea. She slept for twenty-four hours and was then all right.

W.R. has had relapsing-remitting MS since 1997, characterized by six attacks in nine years. Since starting Copaxone right after the first attack she has had five relapses, two of which required steroid treatment. W.R. illustrates the good result when disease-modifying medication is started early in the course. She gives herself a subcutaneous injection every day without trouble. She has no injection-site reactions and no other side effects. She calls herself "a poster child" for the management of MS with immuno-modulatory therapy, which will be discussed more thoroughly in chapter 6.

What Is a Disability?

Unfortunately, there is no universal language that doctors, scientists, and researchers speak when it comes to addressing disability. Therefore, many discussions of disability and the course of MS are misleading.

The International Federation of Multiple Sclerosis Societies (IFMSS) is attempting to establish a standard for international studies. But it has been difficult for experts to agree on exactly what is a disability. For example, if a person is in a wheelchair, does that person have a disability? Some say yes. Some say no, if that person remains gainfully employed with an unaltered quality of life. The World Health Organization (WHO) evaluates the person's neurological impairment and distinguishes between the words *disability* and *handicap*. *Disability*, according to the WHO classification, measures difficulties in carrying out daily activities such as dressing and cooking, and *handicap* measures the effects of a disease on occupation and income.

The Disability Status Scale

Most disability scales used in the United States today only measure physical impairment and the ability to walk. The most widely used scale in MS is the Kurtzke Disability Status Scale (Kurtzke, 1961), which measures ten levels of impairment. (In 1983, the Kurtzke DSS was updated by adding 0.5 grades, making twenty steps in all.)

The primary benefit of the DSS lies in measuring disability during clinical studies. Although this scale is not perfect, and scientists continue to seek better ways, it serves as an accepted standard in testing treatments and therapies. The scale is as follows:

1. No disability, minimal signs (Babinski, minimal finger-to-nose ataxia, diminished vibration sense).
2. Minimal disability (slight weakness or stiffness, mild disturbance of gait or mild visuomotor disturbances).
3. Moderate disability (monoparesis, mild hemiparesis, moderate ataxia, disturbing sensory loss, or prominent urinary or eye symptoms, or combinations of lesser dysfunctions).
4. Relatively severe disability not preventing ability to work or carry on normal activities of living, excluding sexual dysfunction. This includes the ability to be up and about twelve hours a day.

5. Disability severe enough to preclude working, with maximal motor function walking unaided up to 500 meters.
6. Assistance (canes, crutches, braces) required for walking.
7. Confined to wheelchair (able to wheel self and enter and leave chair alone).
8. Confined to bed but with effective use of arms.
9. Totally helpless, bedridden patients.
10. Death due to multiple sclerosis.

This scale clearly has its shortcomings. First, some read it to suggest a typical progression of the disease from number 1 to 2, then 2 to 3, and so on to death. As our case studies in chapter 4 show, this is not the case at all. Also, there are many exceptions to the scale. For example, many people who require a cane for walking may be active and working and only have a mild disability, yet their 6 DSS rating doesn't accurately reflect this.

How bad will a disability be? No doctor can really say. It depends totally on how the symptoms affect the individual. If adjustments are made to accommodate MS, there doesn't have to be any disability at all. Disability, in our definition, is really the mismatch of a person's ability and a specific goal. Weakness or spasticity in the legs may interfere with the twenty-six mile marathon, but it will never ruin a good game of poker.

Although there are no guarantees about any individual's prognosis, those who adjust best are those who focus on ability, not disability. A review of case histories shows that, first, time is on the patient's side. And, second, despite a diagnosis of MS, the quality of life can be of the highest standards, provided that the individual doesn't ruin precious periods of remission and stability by focusing on "what ifs" and "worst case" scenarios that will probably never happen.

5

Taking Control

Multiple sclerosis is the most unpredictable of neurological diseases, with symptoms and signs present one day and gone the next. They can even disappear from one hour to the next. A person who can't work in the morning may be well in the evening, and sometimes it's just the opposite. Is this phenomenon just another MS puzzle? Maybe so, but it is one the person with MS can start to solve. There are many explanations for a lot of symptoms, even attacks.

Let's think back to some of the case studies presented in the last chapter. K. S. did not have any MS attacks in six years, but "after starting a new gym exercise routine and playing tennis, he experienced tingling in his left arm and left leg." B. B. also went without a single attack for six years, but "after a bout with . . . hepatitis . . . she developed dizziness, loss of balance, and double vision," which lasted five days. K. L., "while running down an incline on a slippery surface, . . . slipped and fell. The trauma brought on a new attack." T. B. "adopted a baby and was exhausted from the change in routine. [She developed] double vision, dizziness, loss of balance, numbness, and weakness in all four limbs."

Today we know that many factors can affect or aggravate MS. While some will influence the coming and going of symptoms, others will influence the course of the disease and the occurrence of new attacks. Some are even associated with onset.

In this chapter, we'll discuss:

1. Temperature changes
2. Physical exertion and fatigue
3. Virus and other infections
4. Vaccinations
5. Injuries
6. Surgical operations and anesthesia
7. Pregnancy
8. Emotional stress
9. Contraception
10. Weight
11. Miscellaneous influences

Not all people with MS will be affected by all of the aggravating factors. Some people will never be affected by any of them. But why tempt fate? Learning about these factors is the first vital step in taking control.

Temperature Changes

Heat is one of the most common of the aggravating factors known today. But doctors and patients weren't always armed with this information. In the 1930s doctors actually thought that heat was beneficial to MS patients, and many prescribed a fever treatment with a heat box. Since doctors knew of the higher incidence of MS away from the equator, they used to advise patients in northern climates to move to warmer ones. This only led patients from the refrigerator into the fire. Today we know that elevating the body temperature just one degree Fahrenheit, either from outside heat or fever from an infection, can cause new signs to appear or old signs to reappear—temporarily. In fact, because practically no other neurological disease reacts this way, heat was once used as a way to diagnose MS. The "hot bath test" was used to check for changes in vision or for the appearance of the Babinski sign.

Often those with MS will figure out the effects of heat themselves, relating such incidents as, "I was sunbathing at the beach, and after about an hour of lying in the sand, my vision went out in my right eye just like it did last year. I went home, turned on the air conditioner, and two hours later I was back to normal." Or, "In the middle of taking a hot shower, my right leg gave way, just like three months ago. When I got out, I could only drag my leg. But one hour later it was back to normal."

What causes this kind of temporary dysfunction? The best explanation is that a set of nerve fibers has a spot of myelin damage from the past. Nerve conduction recovered, but the myelin never completely repaired itself. When the body is overheated, conduction is slowed, and the nerve impulse traveling down this set of fibers cannot jump the gap where the myelin is damaged. The part of the body supplied by that bundle of nerves stops functioning temporarily until the nerve tract cools off.

There is some question as to whether excessive heat can actually bring on a new attack. It probably can when heat is due to a high fever but not when it is due to exposure to outside heat. Nevertheless, it's a good policy for MS patients in an attack, or those with residual damage, to avoid exposure to excessive heat from such sources as sunbathing, steam baths, saunas, hot tubs, hot showers, and being outside during the hottest part of a summer day. It is probably acceptable for a patient who has completely recovered from an attack and is in remission to continue these activities. (However, because sunbathing is damaging and dangerous to the skin, it's not recommended for anyone—with or without MS.) Those in a slowly progressive stage with permanent residual damage should always avoid exposure to excessive heat.

Managing excessive heat is not impossible. During hot summer days, some patients take aspirin. They have reported that this prevents such symptoms as fluctuation in vision. Simply soaking the legs in cold water is enough to lower temperature. Depending on the geographical location, an air-conditioning unit may be necessary. (Check with your accountant; it may be tax deductible.)

Excessive cold can also be a bad influence on MS. Although cold packs have long been recognized as an effective part of physical therapy in treatment of spasticity, excessive exposure to cold weather can make walking more difficult by aggravating muscle stiffness.

PHYSICAL EXERTION AND FATIGUE

Physical exhaustion is another common aggravator of MS. It can not only make an old symptom worse but can bring on an attack of symptoms never present before. A typical situation is described in this patient's account: "I had gotten well from weakness in my left leg. I was in Hawaii and started playing tennis again. One day during a heavy tennis match both legs became so weak they could no longer hold me up. I had to be helped off the tennis court. I went to bed, and the weakness was better the next day, but it took a full week to completely clear up."

The patient had no history of weakness in the right leg, so this was a new attack—and it was brought on by physical exertion.

Many people with MS want to know if too much sexual activity is considered overexertion. This is not a significant factor, nor is the rise in temperature during sex. The only time sex may be too much of an exertion is when the person has weak legs. In this case, some positions in sexual intercourse are better than others.

Fatigue can also lead to a new attack. This is commonly seen in people who overwork or overplay. This precipitation of symptoms by fatigue is so universal in MS that most authorities now treat new attacks with rest at least as the first measure. A new attack of leg weakness will often pass with just two days of bed rest.

Virus and Other Infections

Infections, especially virus infections, are likely to precipitate new MS attacks as well as aggravate old symptoms. Viral influenza is the worst offender; during flu epidemics neurologists see many of their MS patients. Many studies show increase in MS attacks during the months when respiratory infections are common.

Infections and viruses precipitate attacks because they stimulate the immune system to put out antibodies. In the process the immune system may also put out antimyelin antibodies. Additionally, infection can cause worsening due to accompanying high fever.

Avoiding colds, sore throats, and especially the flu are important measures in staying free of new MS attacks. This can be done first by maintaining resistance through good nutrition and the proper amounts of rest and sleep. Although the effectiveness of vitamin C is controversial, it can't hurt to use it. Whenever possible, sick people during flu epidemics should be avoided.

Surprisingly enough, current medical evidence suggests that the most effective way to combat colds and flus is simply to wash the hands. Scientists recently discovered that most colds and flu infections are spread not by airborne viruses but by viruses that are picked up on the hands and transferred to the nose or eye ducts. A thirty-second hand washing can rid the skin of 90 percent of particles carrying viruses.

It isn't necessary to shake someone's hand to pick up a virus. Viruses can be picked up from doorknobs, computer terminals, or public telephones. This is not to suggest that anyone turn into a germ-fanatic Howard Hughes, but washing the hands more frequently during flu season is prudent. Also during the flu season, it's best not to use hand lotion, because bacteria and viruses can colonize in the lotion.

Doctors, nurses, dentists, or lab technicians should not touch anyone without washing their hands. This is true even in the sterile environment of a hospital. Researchers at the Centers for Disease Control in Atlanta estimate that more than 100,000 people a year actually die either directly or indirectly from infections they acquire in hospitals. How many more get hospital-acquired infections and don't die has not been reported.

At one hospital, urinary tract infections were cut in half by requiring doctors, nurses, and aides to wash their hands after emptying catheter bags. To cut similar risks, ask all medical personnel to wash their hands. You might feel a bit uncomfortable doing this, but a little embarrassment is certainly worthwhile if it prevents an MS relapse.

Local infections, such as boils, abscesses, and infected cuts and burns have also been known to activate the onset symptoms of MS. It is always wise to have boils and abscesses treated by a doctor as soon as possible. Do not attempt to treat them yourself. Cuts and burns should be kept as clean as possible. (This means not peeking under sterile bandages and asking the doctor if antibiotics are recommended to prevent secondary infection.)

VACCINATIONS

One clear dilemma for people with MS is whether or not to get a flu shot during an epidemic. It might seem like an obvious preventative measure, but vaccinations have in the past been associated both with first attacks of MS and with new attacks in established MS cases. This is not surprising, since the purpose of a vaccine is to stimulate the immune system to develop antibodies against disease.

The association between flu shots and MS attacks, however, has only been reported in case studies and has not been confirmed in studies of large groups of patients. A UCLA MS Clinic study, for instance, showed that no MS patients had exacerbations following immunization with swine flu vaccine. Still, some neurologists believe, based on anecdotal evidence, that vaccinations can be risky for people with MS. I personally do not recommend the flu vaccine for those in complete remission. I will, however, recommend it for patients with disability, since the risk of getting the flu outweighs the risk of the vaccine. Pharmaceutical alternatives include the drug amantadine (Symmetrel) and Tamiflu, which are often effective in preventing the flu.

Smallpox vaccinations may be dangerous for people with any nervous system disorder, including MS. Since smallpox has been eliminated from the world, this is no longer an issue. For all other types of immunization, such as what's needed when a person is exposed to hepatitis or must travel to a country where cholera or yellow fever exists, the person with MS should probably be vaccinated. But it's not a bad idea to participate actively in the decision. For example, if cholera shots are recommended for travel and not necessarily required, the patient should research when the last epidemic occurred and find out if cholera is currently active in his or her destination. Then the patient and doctor can reasonably weigh the risks. Finally, if there has been even a hint of exacerbation following a vaccination in the past, future vaccinations should be avoided.

Injuries

The exact relationship of injuries to onset of MS has long been debated. The patient will naturally try to relate onset to a definable incident. Many case studies are very convincing—injuries are dramatic events that will easily be remembered by patients—but they are not truly valid statistical evidence.

McAlpine believed, "Trauma to a limb or any part of the body, slight or severe, including operations, may occasionally precipitate the disease in a predisposed person or cause a relapse."

In a 1972 study of 250 MS patients, McAlpine's researchers found that 14 percent had an injury within three months prior to onset. In a parallel study of 250 patients with other diseases, only 5.4 percent had an injury within three months prior to onset. Although the studies showed a significant difference, most authorities do not believe that injury actually causes MS. It is more likely that injury brings out symptoms of an existing lesion that was previously silent.

Scientists do agree, however, that an injury can trigger a new attack. Often the attack is localized in the area that has been injured. One patient, in complete remission and without symptoms, got up from bed in the middle of the night to go to the bathroom and stubbed his right toe on a chair. At first he had pain only in the toe. But the next morning there was numbness and tingling in the right foot, which spread up the right leg to waist level over the next twenty-four hours. That wasn't a particularly serious attack, but neither was the injury. More serious injuries can have more serious results.

When the injury is the patient's fault there is little to resolve. But when the injury is caused by another person, directly or indirectly, tough legal questions are raised. I have been involved in several lawsuits in which patients stood to gain a lot by proving the injury triggered a new attack or made existing MS symptoms permanently worse. The key element in such cases is the time sequence. If an injury is followed by a new MS attack or a worsening of old damage within two or three weeks, it may be accepted as the precipitating factor. A delay of a month or more casts doubt on the injury as a precipitant for the attack.

One patient, in complete remission, was in an auto accident in which she hit her head and was knocked unconscious. This was followed a few days later by loss of vision in both eyes and weakness in the legs. The damage improved, but she never fully recovered. She won a large award in court.

Another patient who was injured in an auto accident had new MS symptoms three months later. This longer delay was the main factor in the patient's loss of the lawsuit and failure to collect damages.

Interestingly, the Veterans Administration has a policy of accepting MS as a service-related illness if onset occurs within seven years after discharge from the service.

Still, it should be emphasized that the triggering of a new attack by an injury is a rare occurrence and not an explanation for most MS attacks. In many cases the question is, Which came first, the injury or the MS attack? Sometimes an injury is the result of the patient's neurological difficulty, not the cause. If a patient falls down the steps and experiences an attack, was the fall the first symptom of the attack or the precipitating factor? This, as seen in many workers' compensation and personal injury cases, is difficult to discern.

Nevertheless, the moral of this story is that avoiding injury is an important measure in keeping MS quiet. The following checklist includes some guidelines:

1. Wear your seat belt and drive defensively.
2. Study your home for such hazards as a crack in the front step, a carpet seam that's fraying, an unstable bookshelf and so on. Don't put off repairs.
3. Make sure all stairways have railings, and use them.
4. Outside the home, always be on the lookout for water puddles, oil and grease spots, and stretches of ice.
5. Wear shoes with good heels and soles. Worn shoes have no gripping power and make it easy to slip and fall. Sand the bottoms of new shoes a little so they're not slippery.
6. Use a night-light in your bedroom, or make sure you're in the habit of turning on the lights when getting up in the middle of the night.
7. Make sure all children's toys are put away after use.
8. Take your time. Rushing is a common cause of accidents. Missing the first few minutes of a play is far less significant than the consequences of an injury.
9. Tranquilizers, sleeping pills, alcohol, and antihistamines affect balance; be extra careful when using them.

SURGICAL OPERATIONS AND ANESTHESIA

Since the two go hand in hand, it is difficult for researchers to distinguish the effects of surgery from the effects of anesthesia. But it is fairly common for surgery to be followed by a new attack within one or two weeks. The cause is usually thought to be stress on the immune system, but other factors such as emotional stress may also play a part. In one study 8 out of 40 MS patients gradually deteriorated after a hysterectomy. The results are inconclusive because of the small size of the study, and investigators believe some hormonal or psychological factors might also be involved.

Although it has never been proved that surgery affects the course of the disease, avoiding unnecessary operations is a good principle for everyone to follow. When surgery is necessary, be sure the surgeon and anesthesiologist consult with the neurologist. They will need to discuss precautions such as preventing the fever that is very common after surgical procedures.

Spinal anesthesia should be avoided; this may precipitate an MS relapse. General or local anesthesia is a better choice. Local anesthesia is especially well tolerated by people with MS. In a 1978 study of 98 patients who had more than 1,000 local anesthetics for minor operations and dental work, only 4 noticed deterioration during the following month.

Pregnancy

Whether or not to plan a family is a frequent question for women with MS, particularly because the disease often begins during child-bearing years. At one time pregnancy was thought to be a danger to the MS patient, but the latest thinking is that it is not. Some researchers believe that pregnancy, which suppresses the immune system, may temporarily improve MS.

In early 1987 the highly sensational "Baby M" trial brought much misinformation about MS and pregnancy into the headlines. The case involved a New Jersey couple, Elizabeth and William Stern, who hired a surrogate mother to have a child for them. The surrogate mother later went to court to gain custody of the child. Mrs. Stern, a practicing pediatrician, claimed that she could not bear her own children because she had had “a mild form” of multiple sclerosis since 1979. In widely reported court testimony, a neurologist testified on her behalf that a woman suffering from multiple sclerosis would be playing medical “Russian roulette” if she chose to bear children. He said that a pregnancy could have jeopardized Mrs. Stern’s health, possibly resulting in paralysis.

This court testimony did a great disservice to women with MS who are considering having a family. Study after study has shown that pregnancy has no effect on subsequent MS disability. A study published in the August 1986 issue of *Neurology* compared 178 women with no pregnancies, one pregnancy, or two or more pregnancies. All had clinically definite MS. There was no difference in long-term disability. Interestingly, women who had MS onset during pregnancy had less disability and less MS activity than those with onset before or after pregnancy.

Some early studies have shown an increased frequency in exacerbations in the first three to six months after the birth of a baby. This increase in incidence is not necessarily due to the pregnancy but more likely to the physical exertion involved in caring for a newborn. The mother is up all night, the comfortable daily routines are interrupted, and a new baby in the house can be exhausting. (When T. B. became my patient, I wasn’t surprised to learn that she had had an attack soon after bringing the new baby home—even though her baby was adopted.)

My advice to women with MS who want to have children is to have someone help them out for the first six weeks after giving birth. This will greatly lower the risk of an attack.

Many patients fear they will transmit MS to their children. At the present time there is no scientific evidence that MS is transmitted from parent to child. However, there may be a transmission of *susceptibility* to MS.

A type of antigen—HLA—has been shown to have an increased incidence in MS patients and close family members. Some have suggested this antigen indicates an increased risk of developing MS later in life. But at this point genetic science tell us that MS cannot be transmitted to a baby and that inheritance remains only a minor suspect as the cause of the disease. The incidence of parents and children both having MS is very rare. Also, anyone desiring a family today has many reasons to be optimistic that a cure for MS will be available by the time the next generation reaches the average age of MS onset.

The decision to start a family should be based on the disability level at the time of discussion, the ability to care for children in later years, and the ability to deal with the stress of raising a family.

Emotional Stress

Stress is the most debatable of all the possible aggravating factors of MS. Some people with MS attempt to relate every attack to an emotional crisis.

The notion that both onset and deterioration of MS follow emotional trauma or nervous strain has been widely discussed for more than a century. A historical account from the diary and letters of Sir Augustus Frederick d'Este, now kept in the library of the Royal College of Physicians in London, reads in part:

> *In the month of December 1822 I traveled from Ramsgate to the Highlands of Scotland for the pur-*

> *pose of passing some days with a Relation for whom I had the affection of a son. On arrival I found him dead. I attended his funeral; there were many persons present and I struggled violently not to weep: I was however unable to prevent myself from doing so. Shortly after the funeral I was obliged to have my letters read to me and their answers written for me, as my eyes were so attacked that when fixed upon minute objects indistinctness of vision was the consequence. Until I attempted to read, or to cut my pen, I was not aware of my eyes being in the least attacked. Soon after I went to Ireland, and without anything having been done to my eyes, they completely recovered their strength and distinctness of vision.*

Many patients have attacks related to emotional crisis or stress. But in many situations the emotional upset is the first symptom of a new attack, not the cause. Often an attack is heralded by mood change or emotional lability. A research team from the University of Alberta in Edmonton, Canada, studied forty MS patients and recently reported that those in exacerbation perceived their stresses to be far greater than the others. Drs. Kenneth and Sharon Warren, the husband-and-wife team behind this study, raise the question of whether stress precipitates the attack or whether the patient building up to an attack has a greater reaction to stress and is less able to cope with it.

In March, 2004, three investigators published a report online in the *British Medical Journal* on a forty-year summary of medical literature on the possibility of a link between stress and MS. This meta-analysis, which combined statistics from fourteen of the papers, did note a significant increase in the risk of relapse after stressful or traumatic life events.

But, since the individual studies varied in protocols, and relied on long-term recollections of the subjects, there were no definitive answers. In the end, the authors called for a clinical trial.

The bottom line is that stress is a part of normal life and should not be avoided. It is unfortunate when a doctor tells a family that stress can trigger new attacks and the patient is then treated with kid gloves. This can lead to a neurotic patient's manipulating family and friends. This kind of unhealthy relationship has a worse overall effect on the person with MS than stress ever will.

It may be advisable for the person with MS to seek psychotherapy for emotional stress. For best results, the psychotherapy should be focused on specific problems in the patient's life, such as marriage or career, but not MS. MS may be an added burden to bear, but it should not be used as an excuse to mask problems that have little to do with the disease.

Depression

MS researchers have found an increase in the statistics for major depression among people with MS—50 to 60 percent will suffer depression at some point in their lifetime, as opposed to about 17 percent of those without the disease. University of Toronto researchers have recently found structural changes in the brain, using magnetic resonance imaging, and compared the brains of 21 people with MS and depression to 19 people with MS and no depression. Those with depression did show more signs of lesions and atrophy, but not in every case. It is now generally accepted that in some patients depression can be caused by MS, not just be a reaction to it. While researchers continue to investigate, it's important to remember that there are many effective new treatments for depression, and a mental health expert should be added to the management team as needed.

Contraception

At one time the birth control pill was thought harmful to MS patients, and at another time it was thought to be beneficial. Actually, it is neither. A large study showed no evidence that the pill caused any increased disability over a duration of time. If it is recommended by a gynecologist and well tolerated by the patient, it can be used.

Use of some other birth control methods, such as the diaphragm, contraceptive sponge, or condom, may present difficulties for those with incoordination of hands, although many partners find assisting with them an enjoyable part of sexual foreplay. Intrauterine devices (IUDs) are not recommended for patients with numbness or decreased sensitivity in the pelvic area since they may not be able to identify slippage of the device.

Weight

In general, weight will not affect MS, although being too overweight may aggravate such symptoms as weak legs and bowel problems. It can also create serious health problems unrelated to MS, such as heart disease, diabetes, and high blood pressure. This can not only impair the quality of life but may complicate treatment of MS if medications conflict. Everyone should watch his or her weight and keep as fit as possible. For the wheelchair-bound, a reduction in daily calorie intake is important to compensate for the decrease in the amount of calories burned.

Being underweight also has its problems. It often signals a lack of good nutrition, which can lower immunity and make the person with MS more susceptible to flu and cold viruses.

Miscellaneous Influences

Menstruation

Menstruation is generally not considered an aggravating factor in MS. In fact, a 1952 study showed a definite tendency toward improvement during menstruation and during the first half of the menstrual cycle. In rare cases preexisting emotional lability might be temporarily aggravated.

Smoking

Although smoking can cause other problems and diseases, it is not known to aggravate any particular feature of MS.

Drugs

Alcohol will aggravate some existing problems, but only temporarily. The use of alcohol in moderation is not harmful, but the person with MS should recognize its side effects. Alcohol can cause mild balance disorders, so those with this preexisting symptom should drink less. Since alcohol causes urinary frequency, those with bladder control trouble will have aggravation of symptoms. A person with weak legs may tend to have swelling of the feet. In addition, alcohol might cause dizziness, lightheadedness, or fainting.

Marijuana, cocaine, and other drugs have the same effects on the person with MS—no better, no worse—as on the general population.

Coffee and Tea

Caffeinated beverages are valuable stimulants in everyday life, but they will aggravate urinary frequency and urgency and can aggravate hand tremors in patients with preexisting symptoms. For many other people with MS, however, coffee and tea are the safest of any stimulants used to combat afternoon fatigue.

Learning to lessen the risk of new attacks and to prevent worsening of old symptoms is up to the patient. Some people won't give up baking on the beach—no one's going to tell *them* there's something they can't do! This is not unique to people with MS, either. We've all seen an out-of-shape dad trying to beat his teenage son in a one-on-one basketball game. Basically, he's refusing to adjust gracefully to the reality of getting older. We all have to adjust to one thing or another, so don't be stubborn and do your best to avoid the factors known to aggravate MS. In the long run, you'll save yourself greater adjustments.

6

Best Treatments to Beat MS

Changing the Course

Until the cause of MS is proved, treatment cannot be truly scientific. This doesn't mean that many treatments today aren't effective. It just means that because MS is still a mystery disease, many treatments may be disputed now or in the future.

The tendency of MS to remit, or improve spontaneously, makes it very difficult for scientists and patients to evaluate various treatments. In fact, this characteristic of MS has led to many ineffective, even bizarre treatments, not to mention a host of false claims for a cure. It is important to accept that today there is no cure for multiple sclerosis.

But new advances can modify the course of the disease, lessen the frequency and severity of attacks, manage symptoms, and improve the quality of life for people with MS and their families.

We've come a long way since 1884 when Charcot, the pioneer of MS treatment, had tried gold chloride, zinc sulfate, strychnine, silver nitrate, electrical stimulation, belladonna, ergot, potassium bromide, and hydrotherapy. When all was said and done, he admitted that none of the results had been very favorable.

Later, as various causes of MS were suspected, different treatments came into vogue. When infection was first being evaluated, "anti-infectious agents" were tried on many patients. A typhoid vaccine was used to induce fever therapy and a heat box was used to raise the body temperature to kill the suspected spirochetal disease. Today we know that raising body temperature and inducing fever have negative effects on MS patients, but before 1935 there was a belief that "you have to get worse before you get better." Other early treatments that fell by the wayside include dietary tonics and stimulants, neurosurgery, dental and tonsil extraction, ultraviolet light, and hypnosis. More recent treatments that have failed include massive vitamin therapy, the hyperbaric (high-pressure) oxygen chamber, chelation, and others.

How do we know which treatments are of little or no value? First, they don't stand the test of time. If they were effective, they wouldn't fall by the wayside from year to year. Second, they don't hold up to scientific scrutiny. Basically there is only one proper way to evaluate a proposed treatment—a double-blind control study. A double-blind control is a study in which two groups of patients are started in a program at the same time. One group gets the treatment and the other gets a placebo—an inactive pharmaceutical substance given to compare the effect of the "real" treatment on trial. Neither the patient nor the doctor knows who got the real treatment and who got the placebo until the end of the study.

One problem with this type of study, especially in MS, is that the patient getting the placebo is often helped because of the psychological effect of believing that something positive is being done. Some patients in a clinical environment away from the stresses of everyday life, who might even bask in the attention that comes with good medical care, will report they feel better after taking the placebo. This is called a "placebo effect" and it has been known to influence up to 70 percent of MS patients in clinical trials. While this can really confuse test results, the double-blind study is still the only scientifically acknowledged test today. For this very reason, many MS treatment studies do not follow the double-blind protocol.

Some researchers are also forced to sidestep double-blind studies because of difficulties in finding participants. Many patients do not want to enter a prolonged program without a guarantee they will be getting the real treatment. It is difficult to ask people with an incurable disease to give their time, their hopes, and their energies just to advance science. Compassion often hangs in the balance against science. If a study is of a truly promising treatment for MS, doctors may proceed without a double-blind control rather than deprive a patient of a drug that might work. In other cases willing participants are rejected from a study because of involvement in previous tests, a factor that could alter results. In fact, because of the enormous amount of clinical trials being conducted, many researchers are complaining that too many of the eligible candidates have already been "taken."

Treatments for New Attacks

When dealing with a new attack, three treatments have stood the test of time: rest, steroids, and treatment of underlying infection.

Rest

The onset of new symptoms should be reported to the doctor, who will determine whether the symptoms are MS-related or not. If a new attack is beginning, resting at home is the best treatment. How much rest depends on the seriousness of the attack. In some attacks of weak legs, you should get off your feet for a few days. For numbness or tingling, take rest periods during the day, and avoid exercise or overexertion. With a visual attack, rest, avoid excessive heat, and smoking and drinking. (Smoking and drinking have not been definitely shown to worsen an attack, but you don't want to pass up any bets.) Rest the eyes by avoiding reading and television.

Rest is often very effective in shortening the attack. In twenty-seven years of personal experience, I have found that rest at the beginning of an attack can often bring a person out of that attack within a few days.

Steroid Treatment

If an attack is more serious or symptoms have gone on for two weeks or more, steroid (cortisone) treatment may be prescribed. This can be accomplished by giving ACTH (adrenocorticotrophic hormone), a protein hormone extracted from the beef pituitary gland that stimulates cortisone output by the adrenal gland. ACTH was actually proved effective in a double-blind study by a national research committee in 1970, headed by Augustus Rose, the late professor emeritus at UCLA.

In the past ACTH has been given intravenously, generally in the hospital, but an intramuscular gel now makes hospitalization unnecessary. Synthetic steroids, such as prednisone and prednisolone, can be used orally and thus are used more commonly than ACTH. They have never really been tested scientifically but are considered effective based on successful double-blind ACTH studies.

Two different mechanisms are at work with steroids. First, steroids decrease antibody production by the immune system.

If a "bad" antibody is at work, as current theories suggest, steroids may bring the patient out of the attack quickly. Second, steroids act locally to reduce the swelling and inflammation of myelin. They may improve nerve conduction in the demyelinated area by chemical changes such as increasing the nerve cell's potassium and decreasing the sodium levels.

Steroid treatments, both oral and injected, have both favorable and unfavorable effects. They don't always work. They are more likely to work on optic neuritis, brain stem symptoms such as double vision and facial weakness, and spinal cord symptoms in which spastic weakness is the main problem. They work less well for purely sensory attacks and for cerebellar attacks such as tremor, incoordination, and loss of balance. Dramatic effects are seen more commonly in MS cases of fewer than five years. Response to steroid treatments is less dramatic later in the course.

Common side effects found in the short-term use of steroid treatments include increased appetite, weight gain, water retention, nervousness, and insomnia. Less common side effects, unlikely to occur except with prolonged use, include:

1. Lower resistance to infection, such as activation of dormant tuberculosis. If the patient has a history of TB, anti-TB drugs should be used.
2. Loss of mineral content from bones, making the patient susceptible to fracture.
3. Interference with blood supply to certain joints, especially the hip joint. A rare complication known as *aseptic necrosis* results in the disintegration of the hip or shoulder joint.
4. Cataracts, reported after years of prolonged use.
5. Changes in sex hormone levels that result in excess hair growth on the face, arms, and legs, and interference in menstruation.

6. Aggravation of latent diabetes or worsening of controlled diabetes.
7. Severe acne.
8. Thin, fragile skin with easy bruising.
9. Impaired wound healing.
10. Increased sweating.
11. Occasional psychiatric breaks, hallucinations, or delusions.
12. Convulsions.
13. Euphoria, a false sense of well-being that can cause confusion in the evaluation of whether or not steroids are indeed beneficial to the patient. The patient may report a dramatic improvement although the examination shows no change.
14. Increased secretion of stomach acid, which can aggravate and cause bleeding in a preexisting stomach ulcer. If the patient has a history of ulcers, antacids or ulcer drugs should be taken.
15. Rise in blood pressure.

A typical state in those who stay on steroid treatment for a long period of time is called the Cushingoid state, named for Dr. Harvey Cushing. It includes a moon face, a prominent dowager's hump at the lower neck and upper back, and purple streaks on the skin of the abdominal wall.

This list of possible side effects should *not* frighten patients away from these very valuable drugs. In situations where they have to be used in long treatment, therapy every other day seems to help avoid bad side effects. And when used in a short course of two to six weeks, the benefits far outweigh the risks. Today, they remain the only quick scientifically proved way out of a new attack, which helps the patient avoid potentially permanent residual damage.

Steroid treatment is used in many diseases, including rheumatic disease, collagen disease, skin diseases, eye diseases, allergies, lung and some gastrointestinal diseases, blood disorders, some infections, and even some cancers.

For MS treatment, steroids are typically given in pill form, starting with a high dose for one or two weeks and then tapering off rapidly or slowly, depending on how severe the attack is and how quickly symptoms disappear. A typical course for ON is two or three weeks; a typical course for spinal cord symptoms is six weeks.

It is not good practice to stop the drugs suddenly if the patient has been using them for more than two weeks, because "steroid withdrawal" may occur. The patient may experience a drop in blood pressure, headaches, blurring of vision, lethargy, dizziness, lightheadedness, fainting, general weakness, and even a flare-up of the attack that was beginning to get better. If, however, the symptoms disappear in one week, the patient may be taken off steroids quickly without side effects.

Treatment of Infection

Frequently infection is at the basis of a new attack. When this is the case, clearing up the infection can get the patient out of the attack quickly. For example, acute sinusitis or a dental abscess can cause an attack of ON. A urinary or bladder infection can cause an attack of weakness and stiff legs. In these cases, antibiotics can effectively treat the attack.

Modifying the Disease Course

One of the most important focuses for MS researchers has been the prevention of further attacks in the relapsing-remitting type and the prevention of worsening in the progressive types. For people with MS, this would, in effect, be a "cure." And great strides have been made in this area in the past few years. As a group, they are called disease-modifying drugs and in individual clinical trials which compared a drug against a placebo, MS attacks were reduced by 28 to 60 percent by different treatments. Most people on the disease-modifying drugs showed fewer, smaller, or no new lesions at all on MRI scans. And, in the opinion of the National MS Society Medical Advisory Board, limiting lesions may be the way to reduce future disability. Here's how this treatment revolution started and where it stands today with six disease-modifying drugs currently approved by the FDA.

How We Got Here

In Israel in the early 1970s, scientists worked on the assumption that myelin basic protein (MBP), which constitutes about 30 percent of myelin, was the "MS antigen" and might induce a tolerance for EAE if injected into animals with the disease. This plan of attack against MS was called immune system desensitization. It is much like an allergist injecting you to build up a tolerance for bee stings or certain pollens. They were investigating the theory that if you inject an "MS antigen," you can build up an immune tolerance. After the tests had some positive results, a synthetic MBP was engineered, called copolymer-1 (COP-1). This worked even better in lab animals. In 1985 a report was presented at the annual meeting of the American Academy of Neurology, based on a two-year double-blind trial of humans tested at Albert Einstein College of Medicine in New York City. Although some experts noted problems with the design of the study, it was believed that daily injections of COP-1 reduced the frequency of attacks. Generally, those on the placebo were reported to have advancement of the disease on the Kurtzke scale, while those taking the drug showed none.

Glatiramer acetate (Copolymer-1, Copaxone)

In 1996, COP-1 was released as Copaxone. This injectable drug was engineered to desensitize the immune system. Although no one knows exactly how it works, it is believed to alter the basic mechanism of T-cell activation. Studies show it reduces the frequency of MS relapses by a third, reduces the number of MS lesions seen on MRI—especially new ones—and may reduce the number of new lesions that evolve into "black holes," areas that cause permanent damage to nerve fibers, called axons.

Approximately 13 percent of patients using Copaxone experience immediate systemic reactions which are transient and include flushing, chest pain or tightness, shortness of breath, palpitations of the heart, and anxiety. Occasionally, lymph node enlargement occurs. The most common side effects are injection-site reactions: pain, redness, thickening of skin, and atrophy of subcutaneous fat. A severe allergic reaction has been documented in only one case. This consisted of two episodes of angioedema: swelling of lip, neck, face, and right foot, requiring emergency treatment, with complete recovery after discontinuation of the drug. Compared to the other drugs, Copaxone is the safest, showing the fewest toxic side effects, but the injection-site reactions are the most troublesome. There is hope that an oral form of the medication will be developed. For the present, it is given by subcutaneous injection daily at a dose of 20mg.

Interferons

The road to today's success with interferon treatment was at first a bumpy one. Interferons are protein substances that are produced naturally in the body by the natural killer cells of the immune system in response to a variety of invaders such as viruses and bacteria. They have antiviral, antiproliferative, and immunomodulatory properties, thus working to counteract infections, tumors, and allergic diseases. It is now apparent that interferon occurs in three forms: alpha, beta and gamma.

In MS research, much knowledge was gained from test results of both alpha and gamma interferon. In 1983–1984, when the cost of alpha interferon was very high, a small double-blind test of MS patients was funded by a million-dollar grant from the National Multiple Sclerosis Society, along with other contributions from the National Institutes of Health, the Leiper Trust, the Hearst Foundation, and the J. M. McDonald Foundation. Researchers set out to find if injections of 5 million units a day of alpha interferon for six months would change the frequency of attacks of MS in twenty-four patients from three medical centers (the University of California at San Francisco, Scripps College, and Stanford University). Unfortunately, design flaws in the study made the results appear less promising than they actually were.

At the 1986 annual meeting of the American Academy of Neurology, gamma interferon probably generated the most excitement of any MS therapy—even though use of the drug proved to be a complete disaster and clinical trials were halted after one month when seven out of eighteen patients experienced acute attacks. Dr. Kenneth Johnson, professor and chairman of the Department of Neurology at the University of Maryland was praised by colleagues for his honesty in reporting the test failure. But there was good reason for the candor—and the excitement. There had never been any kind of therapy that had exacerbated the disease like gamma interferon. In a backhanded way, the study actually supported the theory that modifying the immune system will modify the disease. The results of Johnson's test suggest that if gamma interferon exacerbates MS, an effective treatment might involve tailoring a drug to do the opposite.

Thus beta interferon became the next agent to investigate. In 1991, the National Institutes of Health funded a $2 million clinical trial of beta interferon. It reduced relapse frequency (by about one third) and severity compared with placebo. Disease progression as measured by EDSS was also decreased. And MS lesions on MRI were reduced in number or disappeared.

Betaseron is injected under the skin every other day; Avonex, injected into the muscle weekly; Rebif, injected under the skin three times a week.

Betaseron has now been in use for sixteen years and, studies show, yearly relapse rates decreased up to 40 percent over the control group. Progression of disability was delayed by six years. Conversion to a progressive course was 16 percent lower.

The other interferons have been in use for a shorter time, but also significantly lower annual relapse rates and disability risk. How interferons work has never been fully established. But there is evidence that these agents interfere with T-cell activation, thus inhibiting the body's immune response, and interfere with blood-brain barrier function as evidenced by the dramatic reduction in number of enhanced (new) lesions on MRI seen in many MS patients who receive the drug.

The most commonly reported side effects of interferons are injection-site reactions: pain, redness, bruising, and swelling; rarely, skin necrosis (death of tissue). Other adverse events are flu-like symptoms (muscle pain, fatigue, malaise, headache, fever and chills), elevated liver enzyme levels, mild white blood cell abnormalities, and depression. Flu-like symptoms tend to stop occurring after the first year of use. Concomitant medication (acetaminophen or a nonsteroidal anti-inflammatory drug) can prevent and/or treat these symptoms. The NSAIDs should be used at the time of injection, then several hours later if any flu-like symptoms are noted. Other helpful measures are to build up the interferon dose gradually and early evening dosing (so the person is sleeping when the interferon dose peaks in eight to ten hours). No long-term safety concerns have emerged after sixteen years of treatment with interferon beta medications. However, blood counts, liver function tests, and thyroid function tests should be performed regularly. There is an increased frequency of depression, even suicidal thoughts. Patients should report such symptoms immediately and cessation of therapy should be considered. The effectiveness of interferon beta may be compromised by its potential to produce neutralizing antibodies which can diminish the effect on relapse rates and on MRI measures of disease activity. Thus testing for neutralizing antibodies should be part of the management of MS patients on the interferons.

Natalizumab (Tysabri)

Scientists believe if they can learn either how to turn on cells that are underrepresented or turn off cells that are overrepresented, they'll be able to arrest MS in humans. Investigators in several research laboratories had dramatic results applying this theory to EAE in mice experiments. In January 1985 researchers from Stanford University announced they were able to turn off certain T cells, using a biotechnological advance called monoclonal antibodies. This halted the myelin damage of EAE in 90 percent of the mice within seventy-two hours and reversed early symptoms. In other studies, when mice were injected with anti-T-helper monoclonal antibodies before inducing EAE, the disease was prevented entirely.

What exactly is a monoclonal antibody? A regular antibody is an infection-fighting protein produced by B lymphocytes in response to a foreign invader. The monoclonal antibody is a version made in the laboratory, first developed in 1975 by joining B cells of a laboratory mouse (which produce antibodies for a specific antigen) with tumor cells (because they can reproduce rapidly and in great numbers). When the fused mouse cell is cloned, or identically reproduced in unlimited numbers from a single cell, the result is a monoclonal antibody. The beauty of the monoclonal antibody is that it can be designed to destroy a specific cell, such as the subset of T-helper cells targeted only for myelin, while preserving the rest of the immune system, which is needed to fight other infections (without any T-helper cells, a person could easily die of the flu or pneumonia). Because of its ability to strike a specific target, monoclonal antibody therapy has been given the nickname the Magic Bullet. It must be administered every four weeks intravenously at a registered infusion facility.

Natalizumab is a humanized monoclonal antibody targeted against an antigen that mediates the movement of immune-activated T cells through the blood-brain barrier, an important step in the production of MS. In a two-year natalizumab monotherapy trial, there was a 42 percent decrease in disability progression and a 68 percent reduction in annual relapse rates in the treatment group compared with the control group. In a combination study of natalizumab and interferon beta-1A (Avonex) there was a 54 percent reduction in the rate of relapses and a 24 percent decrease in disability progression in patients receiving both compounds compared with those only on Avonex. MRI results were also striking: natalizumab produced an 89 percent reduction in the number of gadolinium-enhanced lesions in both studies.

The FDA approved natalizumab in December 2004 based on available one-year interim data. However, three months later, the drug was withdrawn because of reports that two patients on the natalizumab-plus-beta inferon group developed progressive multifocal leukoencephalopathy (PML), a brain disease caused by a virus. One of the patients died as a result, the other developed severe neurological disabilities.

Shortly thereafter it was reported that a clinical trial patient who had received natalizumab infusions for the treatment of Crohn's disease developed a fatal case of PML. These three patients were among approximately 3,000 patients receiving natalizumab.

In February 2005 natalizumab was withdrawn from the market pending safety review and agreement on a risk reduction program with the FDA. In March 2006 the FDA Central Nervous System Committee voted to approve reintroduction of the drug for first-line therapy for relapsing-remitting MS. Because of its dangers natalizumab should probably be reserved for patients who have failed or cannot tolerate the interferon betas and glatiramer acetate and failed on or do not want to consider mitoxantrone.

Mitoxantrone (Novantrone)

Mitoxantrone, a synthetic immuno-suppressant anticancer drug, *is the only drug currently approved by the FDA as treatment for secondary-progressive MS*. First approved in 1987 for treatment of adult leukemia, it was cleared for use in patients with secondary-progressive MS, deteriorating relapsing-remitting MS, and progressive-relapsing MS, in 2000. Researchers believe a number of mechanisms are at work: suppression of proliferation of lymphocytes, especially T cells; impairment of antigen action; and blockage of myelin destruction. It may limit or prevent demyelination and reduce axonal loss and atrophy.

Mitoxantrone must be given intravenously (IV) every three months at a medical facility. It is a dangerous drug but should be seriously considered as a rescue therapy by those who are failing high-dose/high-frequency interferon beta and are actively worsening clinically or according to MRI. During therapy patients are continued on a disease-modifying drug, interferon beta or glatiramer.

Adverse events include nausea, blue-green discoloration

to urine or sclera of the eye for twenty-four hours (which is harmless), drop in white blood cell count (associated with increased infection risk), liver function test abnormalities, cardiotoxicity (which can lead to congestive heart failure and death) and acute leukemia (which can be fatal). In a study of 802 patients for five years, 35 (4.4 percent) experienced cardiotoxicity and 1 developed acute heart failure. Two cases of leukemia were observed, resulting in one death. In another study, 3 of 134 patients (2.7 percent) developed leukemia. The risk-to-benefit ratio of mitoxantrone therapy in patients with aggressive form of relapsing-remitting MS (three relapses and a 2-point increase in the disability scale over one year) was studied in 100 patients. Over the next year, the annual relapse rate decreased to 0.03 and the disability scale decreased by 1.2 points. The relapse rate and disability scale remained improved over the following four years but three patients subsequently manifested cardiotoxicity and one patient developed acute leukemia. Because of these dangers some doctors limit the use of mitoxantrone to one year. Other doctors limit the cumulative lifetime dose to a certain amount, which is usually reached within two to three years at the recommended dosage.

So is it worth it? One is willing to accept the risk in secondary-progressive MS and deteriorating relapsing-remitting MS because without it, the MS may progress to the point that the potential toxicities are of lesser concern in comparison to what the disease will do.

Who Should Take What?

None of the disease-modifying drugs is recommended for women who are pregnant or plan to be. Risks are weighed against the benefits of the new treatments.

We recommend newly diagnosed patients with evidence of definite MS start either Copaxone, Betaseron, Avonex, or Rebif right away to prevent further attacks and new MRI lesions. This is true also for cases of relapsing-remitting MS in whom attacks are still occurring. Those with deteriorating relapsing-remitting MS not responding to the above agents and those with secondary-progressive disease that is relentlessly worsening should consider Novantrone or Tysabri, in spite of the dangers of these drugs.

We also recommend that people whose disease has been stable for several years—with no attacks and no worsening—can skip this round of treatments and assess the next round of breakthroughs. In the meantime, just follow our suggestions of how to stay in top physical and emotional form.

For the rest, disease-modifying drugs are seen as an investment in the future. Unfortunately, none of the currently available drugs is approved for those with a primary-progressive course. In those cases, the greatest successes in treatment have been the tackling of individual symptoms. With rare exception, every symptom of MS can be treated, and every single patient improved.

7

Treatment of Symptoms and Rehabilitation

Until a treatment was discovered to alter the course of the disease and reverse it, the best strategy was the management of symptoms and rehabilitation of persisting problems. With the use of medication, physical therapy, psychotherapy, mechanical devices, and good old-fashioned common sense, something can be done to help each and every patient. Treatments may vary with the stage and severity of the disease, but the goal remains the same—to return the patient to normal or as near to normal as possible. Every single symptom can be tackled, and everything that happens in MS is treatable, although some symptoms are more easily treatable than others.

The first step in getting good treatment is selecting the right doctor. This is a doctor who knows MS, will follow the case carefully, and will be available when needed. Does this have to be a neurologist? Probably yes, because only a neurologist has managed enough MS patients to know the wide varieties of the disease, and only a neurologist will be up to date on the latest developments in MS research. When making that first appointment, simply ask the nurse if the doctor is an expert in MS or has a special interest in the disease. Be a wise consumer.

With the simple, mild form of MS characterized by occasional attacks with remission, the patient only needs a good neurologist as a guide. In more complicated, advanced MS, the neurologist may need to call on a variety of experts in other fields. These may include physical medicine specialists, orthopedists, urologists, ophthalmologists, otorhinolaryngologists (ear, nose, and throat specialists), psychotherapists, physical therapists, occupational therapists, speech therapists, and visiting nurses. When other experts are called on, the neurologist should function as a team leader, coordinating efforts and preventing fragmented care.

Trust in your neurologist is essential, so find one with whom you can develop a solid rapport. The patient must also participate in team management, informing the neurologist of plans, problems, side effects of medication, and more. The doctor must make sure, for instance, that the patient is not mixing incompatible drugs, such as some antibiotics and antacids. Remind the neurologist of other medications you're taking. Report any skin reactions, such as redness or a rash. Discuss your plans to become pregnant or to start nursing to avoid dangerous side effects to the fetus or newborn from certain medications. Ask the neurologist if the pharmaceutical company publishes a patient information pamphlet. Find out if your medication is dangerous or ineffective when mixed with one or more alcoholic beverages. In general, be as informed as possible.

As we've emphasized, there is no situation in MS that cannot be improved by effort and careful management. Sometimes it can be as simple as taking the right dose of the right medication. At other times it can be as complex as a prolonged program of physical therapy and efficient planning of daily activities to preserve optimal strength and conserve energy.

Starting with the most common symptoms of MS, here's what can be done in all situations.

Weakness

On either a temporary or permanent basis, weakness is very common. It usually affects one leg, but after many years may involve both. The patient occasionally experiences weakness in one or both hands. (As a symptom, weakness should be distinguished from lack of energy, or fatigue.)

The most common weakness is when one leg feels heavy at the hip and the patient has difficulty lifting the leg later in the day, after too much standing or walking. It is especially evident while stepping up curbs and going up stairs. Less commonly, weakness occurs when the patient lifts the foot. This is evident with the tendency of the foot to drag when the leg is tired.

Newly appearing weakness, occurring in a new attack, often responds to just a few days of rest during which the patient avoids standing and walking as much as possible. If weakness has not subsided in one week, a short course of cortisone is often used and may produce complete recovery in a week or two.

Weakness that has persisted more than a year is treated differently. Here the patient may have great improvement in the use of the leg just by using a walking stick. This takes much of the strain off the weak leg, and the limb doesn't tire as quickly. Although the use of a cane appears to many patients to be a step downward and a bad symbol, it is not necessarily a permanent measure. Often the cane is used only in long walks when the leg is likely to be exhausted and is not necessary for shorter distances. Our experience has been that when the patient with a weak leg uses a cane, he or she can do more and last much longer in daily activities.

When the weakness is at the ankle and bending the foot up becomes difficult, the plastic foot-drop orthosis is very helpful. This device is a very lightweight plastic L-shaped splint that fits inside the shoe and keeps the weak foot bent up when the patient is walking. It completely eliminates dragging of the foot, and it does not weigh down the leg. One small problem is that although the device will be hidden by a pants leg, it will show under a dress or skirt and is impossible to wear with high-heeled shoes.

Knee buckling is very rarely a problem in MS, but if this is the case, the long leg brace, which locks the knee so the leg can't give way, is indicated. More often, however, leg weakness at the hip and ankle is present, making the long leg brace too heavy to support.

Weakness has traditionally been tackled with physical therapy and strengthening exercises. Only a physical therapist experienced in treating MS should treat a patient with leg weakness because therapy, above all, should avoid fatiguing the leg. Because many exercises exhaust weak muscles rather than build them up, it is common to hear patients report, "I go to the physical therapist, but when I leave, I feel weaker than before." A properly trained physical therapist will understand what exercises should be done and when to do them.

Probably the best physical therapy exercises for weakness are done in the water. These hydrotherapy exercises use the benefits of buoyancy. Eliminating the pull of gravity makes it easier to move a weak limb through a fuller range of motion. Also, staying off a weak limb will conserve strength for when it is needed.

Some people have the idea that weakness can be prevented by intensive exercise to build up strength, thereby lessening the chances of severe weakness in the future. This doesn't work. The muscle is weak because the nerve feeding it back in the spinal cord isn't functioning properly. Exercising the muscle won't make the nerve work any better, nor will it prevent a future attack.

Weakness of both legs may become a problem after many years with MS. The usual situation is that the person can walk fairly well with a little support in the morning, but later in the day the legs are so tired that the person may need crutches or even a wheelchair. The best way to handle this difficulty is to understand your limits and organize your activities so that you can take rest periods during the day and avoid prolonged standing and walking. Good planning often makes it possible to avoid the end-of-the-day exhaustion completely and eliminates the need for a wheelchair.

Still, the person whose legs are both weak should have a wheelchair on hand to use on such occasions as going out for a whole day or traveling long distances where too much walking may be necessary, thus avoiding the alternative of staying home. When traveling, plan ahead carefully. Call the airline in advance and ask for a chair to get to and from the plane. When touring, try to drive as close to the destination as possible to conserve your leg strength. This may sound so complicated that it might make you less eager to take trips, but once you have the hang of doing it this way, it becomes an easy routine to follow.

Weakness in the hands is much more rare than leg weakness. When it does occur, the same basic principles of treatment apply. Don't exhaust or overuse the weak hand. Plan activities in order to conserve energy. If weakness is at the wrist, a lightweight splint can be used to help overcome it.

In summary, the treatment of weakness depends on whether it is part of a new attack or is an old weakness. Weakness from a new attack is usually reversible with rest and cortisone. Weakness that has been present for a long time is best treated by conserving strength in the limb or limbs involved. By recognizing limits and using common sense measures to avoid overtiredness, weakness can be greatly diminished. When the patient does not recognize certain limitations, chronic overtiredness can make a temporary situation permanently worse.

SPASTICITY

Spasticity is a situation in which a limb becomes stiffer than normal and does not relax easily. It is more common in the legs than in the arms. It is usually evident only when the person gets up to walk, whereupon the leg stiffens out and is difficult to bend at the knee. This forces the person to walk in a stiff-legged fashion, either scuffing the toes or swinging the leg in an outward circle to avoid scuffing them. Spasticity often accompanies weakness, but one can have spasticity without weakness and weakness without spasticity.

In some ways spasticity is nature's compensation for weakness in the legs, as it may keep the weak leg from buckling at the knee. Occasionally, spasticity is so severe that the limb involved will stiffen out or draw up with any change in position or even at a simple touch. Fortunately, there's very good treatment for spasticity including physical therapy, three effective medications, and relaxation techniques.

Physical therapy is probably most effective in this area of MS. Passive stretching of the involved limb is often successful in relieving spasticity, especially when used with cold packs. Cold is an excellent temporary measure for relaxing the spastic limb. Hydrotherapy is the most effective exercise for relief, combining stretching and cool temperatures.

Medications for spasticity include baclofen, dantrolene,

and diazepam. Relatively free of side effects, baclofen (Lioresal) is the best of the antispasticity drugs. Too high a dose may aggravate weakness, but if this is watched carefully, baclofen can be used on a permanent basis to prevent spasticity effectively. The patient should start with half a tablet three times a day, increasing the dose up to two tablets three or four times a day. If weakness is aggravated, the dose is then reduced. Frequently the medication is only needed temporarily. It can be stopped easily to check if spasticity is still present.

Dantrolene (Dantrium) is also very effective in relieving spasticity but has more side effects. It has a greater risk of causing weakness and has a slight risk of liver and kidney damage. Therefore it is not the drug of first choice in the treatment of spasticity. But in severe cases and when other drugs fail, the patient and doctor should decide if the problem outweighs the risk.

Diazepam (Valium) is a muscle relaxant as well as a tranquilizer and is especially useful if spasticity is a problem at night. Taken at bedtime, the patient doesn't have to worry about the side effect of sleepiness. Smaller doses of Valium should be used in the daytime. Prolonged steady use will create a dependency, and withdrawal symptoms can occur when the drug is removed. It is frequently a depressant and may aggravate balance trouble.

Botox (botulinim toxin), best known as the injectible fountain of youth that helps make wrinkles disappear, is now used by many MS physicians for temporary relief of spasticity. There are seven types of botulinim toxins (A to G). Type A is used for wrinkle relief. Type B is now being used as additional therapy to manage severe stiffness in an isolated area. Botox is believed to block the release of acetylcholine, a chemical that signals muscles to contract. Although oral medications are still the first line of treatment for MS spasticity, Botox is safe and effective and can be repeated as needed.

Relaxation techniques, such as yoga, transcendental meditation, biofeedback, and autohypnosis, have all been successful for some patients. Some patients even report that marijuana has beneficial effects in reducing spasticity.

In severe spasticity cases, where physical therapy, medication, and relaxation techniques have failed, more drastic procedures may be indicated, such as dorsal-column stimulation, injection of phenol into the nerves, and surgery.

Dorsal-column stimulation, successfully used in the past for pain relief, is now also used to reduce spasticity in MS. With this technique a device is implanted directly on the spinal cord, and spasticity is interrupted by electrical stimulation. This is a major surgical procedure that involves some tampering with the spinal cord and the possibility of increased spinal cord damage with prolonged use. Its success remains unproved.

Injection of phenol into one or more nerves of spastic limbs has been used mainly in cases where the aductor muscles of the thighs are so spastic that the legs cannot be pulled apart. These phenol "blocks" usually last about six months.

Finally, in the most severe cases of spastic legs, surgery is sometimes used in which the tight muscles or involved nerve roots are cut. These drastic measures are rarely needed or used in MS but are available for the bedridden patient seeking relief.

Hand Tremor and Incoordination

This symptom becomes apparent when the arm or hand performs actions in a clumsy fashion, sometimes with shaking, slowness, poor rhythm, or an inability to control speed or accuracy of movement. This problem also occurs with the legs and feet, but it is more serious when it involves the hand—greater coordination is required for daily chores like buttoning a sweater or cracking an egg.

Many different medications are available for the different types of hand tremors, and each works in different patients. The neurologist usually has a sequence of medications to try.

Propranolol (Inderal), a medication for high blood pressure, is a very effective treatment for hand tremors that occur when the hand is held out in a fixed position—often called essential tremor or posture-holding tremor. If the MS patient's hand tremor falls into this category, this drug may completely relieve it with relatively few minor side effects. The main problem is that too high a dose can cause tiredness, low blood pressure, and slow pulse, and that it cannot be used by patients with asthma.

Clonidine, a medication also used for high blood pressure, may be effective when propranolol fails to control posture-holding tremor. Clonidine also has more likelihood of controlling head tremor as well as hand tremor. The main drawback is that it can cause too big a drop in blood pressure, producing lightheadedness and even fainting.

Primidone (Mysoline), a medication used to treat epileptic seizures, has been effective in some cases of hand tremor when used alone or with propranolol. The side effects include sleepiness, irritability, and nausea if taken on an empty stomach.

Clonazepam (Klonopin), is another antiseizure drug that may be effective in controlling hand tremor. Side effects include sleepiness and depression.

Amantadine (Symmetrel), originally the antiflu drug, was found to be effective in Parkinson's disease and is now being tried in MS for control of hand tremor. It may also help patients with a lack of energy and an unsteady walk. It is worth trying since it has only a few side effects. When they do occur, they can include swelling of the feet, prominence of small veins in the legs, mental confusion, and depression.

Carbidopa-levodopa (Sinemet), a drug that is very effective in treating Parkinson's disease, rarely helps MS but may be tried to control hand tremor if other drugs fail.

Trihexyphenidyl hydrochloride (Artane), one of the old standard drugs used for Parkinson's tremor, may help tremor of MS if used in high doses. High doses, however, cause dry mouth, memory difficulties, and sometimes confusion.

Isoniazid is used in treatment of tuberculosis, but it is also known to help hand tremor in some MS patients. I have tried this drug with patients without any success.

Besides medications, other measures can be used to control hand tremor. First, try to stabilize the elbow of the arm being used by holding it with the other hand or propping it on the table or dresser when doing such activities as eating, brushing teeth, applying makeup, or writing. This can become second nature.

In more severe tremor cases, surgical procedures are available that are also used in some cases of Parkinson's disease. A small lesion is made in the nucleus deep in the cerebral hemisphere. This may decrease or even completely relieve the tremor, but unfortunately the results show only for a short time. Tremors can return a few months later. Although there is hope that the operation will be perfected to produce more lasting benefits, I do not recommend it for MS patients at this time.

Balance Trouble

When balance trouble is mild, the MS patient can learn to compensate easily by standing and walking with a little wider base and taking short steps rather than long strides.

When the balance trouble is moderate to severe other measures are indicated. Easiest of all is the use of a walking stick, which will not only give the person more security and confidence but is useful in fighting off mad dogs, muggers, and mashers. Throughout Europe, a classic cane is a sign of distinction, often used as a wardrobe accessory by statesmen, nobility, and playboys. In Hollywood, television producer Jay Bernstein, who also managed the careers of Farrah Fawcett, Suzanne Somers, and Cicely Tyson, made the cane his "signature."

Unfortunately, many people with MS view a walking stick as a sign of defeat. If they can manage to get along without it, they certainly will. Stubbornly, they also suffer from added fatigue, exhaustion, and a risk of accidents. This is far too great a price to pay.

In cases where balance trouble is more severe, a four-pronged cane, crutches, or a walker may be necessary. These devices are usually only necessary outside. In the house the MS patient with balance trouble can get by very well using furniture and walls to help with balance, along with appropriately placed grab bars. Grab bars are especially important in the bathroom—in the tub, shower, and next to the toilet. In the shower, a shower seat is also an excellent device.

Physical therapy should also be prescribed to teach the patient how to compensate for balance trouble and difficulties with the activities of daily life. If tailored to the individual, it can be extremely effective.

Miscellaneous Walking Difficulty

Walking difficulties may be due to balance trouble, weakness, spasticity, loss of sensation in the feet, vertigo, and visual troubles. Those underlying problems should be first tackled directly. Then other measures can be taken.

When spasticity creates walking trouble, a specially designed shoe, called a rocker shoe, may help the patient have a totally normal or more normal gait. This shoe was made popular by Carolyn Clawson, a woman with MS who discovered that a pair of clogs received from a friend who brought them from Denmark, helped her walk. Clawson had spent two years in a wheelchair and walked with great difficulty using a cane. At the time she said, "I was reprieved from a prison."

The "Clawson clog" is now available for both men and women with about 6,000 pairs distributed. The rocker shoe is most effective for people with a particular combination of spasticity and muscle weakness. The curved sole of the shoe, which looks much like a clog, brings about knee flexion (bending motion) in a more normal manner. This is also supposed to conserve energy and help reduce fatigue. To benefit from such shoes, however, the patient must have fairly good strength and be able to walk independently. As a general rule (with any consumer product), the rocker shoe is best tried before purchase. If you cannot find the rocker shoe locally, you can contact the largest supplier at 1-208-356-6100. Or write:

Clawson Rocker
c/o New Freedom, Inc.
P.O. Box 428
Rexberg, ID 83440

In conclusion, the patient with walking difficulty probably has the most to gain from physical therapy, the best approach. If the walking difficulty is handled properly, using good therapy, appropriate devices, and common sense to avoid fatigue, it is often possible to improve the situation to the point where the patient walks normally.

Numbness, Tingling, and Other Sensory Symptoms

While these common symptoms usually occur in temporary, short-lived attacks with the patient returning completely to normal, sometimes a patient needs treatment of symptoms and has prolonged periods of unpleasant tingling and burning sensations or tight-band feelings around the trunk or limbs. This problem is not a cause of disability but can be a major annoyance to the patient. If the symptoms become difficult to live with, medications are available for good relief.

Nicotinic acid (niacin, one of the B-complex vitamins) is effective, prescribed in doses of 100-milligram tablets three or four times a day. Two antiseizure drugs, Dilantin and Tegretol, may cause balance trouble if the dose is too high but are safe and effective in small doses for sensory symptoms of MS. Triavil, a combination antidepressant and tranquilizer, is effective, but it is usually only given at bedtime, as it can cause sleepiness.

Face Pain

MS is not usually associated with pain, except for that of trigeminal neuralgia, a condition in about 4 percent of patients. Good treatments are available, so the person does not need to suffer these pains stoically.

Dilantin and Tegretol, the antiseizure medications also used for sensory symptoms, are excellent. Because face pains are often cyclic, occurring for a limited period of time, it is usually possible to get the patient total relief with these drugs and then take him or her off the medication entirely. Pains may stay away for years, but if they return the medication can be used again for a short time, again providing complete relief.

Sometimes, the medications will fail or will be too toxic for an individual to tolerate. In that case, three procedures permanently cure the condition—thermocoagulation, glycerol injections, and, although very rarely used, surgery. Thermocoagulation is a procedure performed under local anesthesia. A wire is inserted and threaded up to a spot at the base of the skull where the sensory nerve to the face originates. The wire is heated and pain fibers are numbed, at the same time leaving intact touch and movement nerves and fibers. The procedure is painless and effective, almost always curing pain.

Glycerol injected into the nerve also selectively numbs pain fibers and leaves other important nerves intact. This treatment has been largely abandoned in favor of either thermocoagulation or surgery.

With surgery, the trigeminal nerve is cut or transposed to a new spot. This surgery, involving an operation at the back of the skull, is almost never needed since one of the above measures usually works.

Visual Symptoms

The two basic forms of vision problems are decreased acuity—blurred or cloudy vision or black areas—and double vision, when the object can also seem to jump or move. The treatment, as with many MS symptoms, depends on the stage of the problem. If it is part of a new attack, visual loss often responds dramatically to a short course of steroids (cortisone), often returning completely to normal. If a problem persists, an ophthalmologist should be consulted to prescribe glasses, magnifying glasses, or special lenses.

Double vision (diplopia) is rarely a permanent residual, but when it occurs, covering one eye with an eye patch, or glasses with a prism or frosted lens on one side, completely eliminates the problem. Nystagmus, or jerky movements of the eye, is treated with use of an eye patch. It is recommended that the patch be used alternately over the left and right eyes.

The rare situation of homonymous hemianopsia, in which vision is lost in the right or left half of each eye, usually recovers completely, but when it persists, the patient can learn to compensate by simply turning the head to the affected side.

Other visual aberrations, such as light sensitivity, may interfere with seeing things clearly. For this and other rare situations, an ophthalmologist will have individual remedies such as recommending yellow lenses to lessen contrast problems.

Vertigo

Vertigo is a sensation of motion, typical of seasickness and often described as spinning, turning, rocking, or floating. At times it may be severe enough to prevent the person from standing or walking. Treatment with medication is generally effective, and if the patient experiences symptoms all day long or for more than a few days, medication can be taken as a preventive measure. Dramamine is the most commonly used medication, although Bonine, Marezine, and Torecan are also effective. Drowsiness is a common side effect of these drugs, especially if taken in high doses. Marezine is given by injection; the other medications are available in tablets.

Transderm Scop is still another effective treatment for vertigo. It is a medicinal patch that is placed on the skin behind the ear. The system is programmed to deliver the medication to the body over three days. Only one disc should be worn at a time. It's important to wash the hands after applying the patch to avoid getting the medication in the eyes; this can cause temporary blurring of vision and dilated pupils.

The most common side effect of Transderm Scop is dryness of the mouth, which occurs in about two-thirds of users. Drowsiness occurs in only about 15 percent. In rare cases confusion, with hallucinations, has been reported.

Speech Problems

Speech problems are not very common but they can be a source of great distress to patients when they do occur. MS speech trouble consists of slurring or jerky rhythm. If part of a new attack, the speech problem may clear on its own but if present for two or three months, a speech therapist is recommended. Both problems may be handled by talking more slowly and concentrating on careful enunciation. But the speech therapist will have a program specifically tailored to the individual problem. Retraining exercises, in which the patient analyzes the problem on audio tapes, often help correct it. The earlier the patient begins to monitor speech problems, the better the prognosis for correction.

Swallowing Trouble

Swallowing trouble is a rare complication of MS. It may be brief in duration or permanent, in which case it is often associated with speech trouble. The patient experiencing the trouble may have to exert extra effort to swallow and may even choke on liquids or solids. The patient with this difficulty should be referred to an ear, nose, and throat specialist. Tests will determine whether the problem is due to incoordination or weakness of the swallowing muscles, and the treatment will depend on which is the cause. If the problem is incoordination, special exercises may solve it. If there is weakness of the swallowing muscles, it may be necessary to use artificial devices or have surgery, but this is very rare.

Bladder Problems

Bladder problems are not uncommon in MS. The most common are frequency and urgency—the patient has to urinate too often and in a hurry. Three good medications relieve symptoms when present for more than a week or two—Pro-Banthine, Ditropan, and Tofranil. Pro-Banthine and Ditropan are antispasmodics that help the bladder work normally by allowing it to fill up to a fuller level before it's ready to squeeze back down and empty. Tofranil is an antidepressant that also works to decrease spasms and bring the bladder back to normal in MS. It has an extra benefit in lifting the mood as well. Some of the side effects of the medications include dry mouth, blurred vision, constipation, and sometimes too much urinary retention. Occasionally sweating is suppressed.

The opposite bladder problem—urinary retention, or the inability to empty properly—is a rare occurrence. When this is only partial, and the problem seems to be hesitation or slowness, a simple exercise can overcomc it. The patient is trained to use the hands to push on the lower abdomen while sitting on the toilet. Any degree of urinary retention should be evaluated by a urologist; it can lead to repeated urinary tract infections that can aggravate MS itself by causing more frequent exacerbations.

If bladder problems do not respond to medication or exercise, a complete bladder-training program may be prescribed. This is very often effective, and only very rarely is it necessary to go further and use catheterization or surgery. A catheter is a device used, either intermittently or constantly, that takes over where bladder muscles fail.

Botox, discussed earlier in the treatment of muscle spasticity, is also showing promise in the management of some urinary symptoms. Injected into the external urinary sphincter, Botox can help relieve urgency, frequency, dribbling, retention, and voiding problems. Botox A has been shown to reduce the need for some catheterizations. A small study showed improved quality of life with no significant adverse effects. As FDA approval has not yet been sought by Allergan, the pharmaceutical company that owns the patent on Botox, the relatively high costs of the treatment are not covered by insurance.

Bladder problems can probably be handled much more simply with a commonsense approach. Empty the bladder before leaving the house. Avoid bladder stimulants such as caffeine drinks, beer, or other alcoholic beverages when not close to a bathroom. Avoid liquids close to bedtime if urgency occurs at night.

BOWEL PROBLEMS

In general, the bowel is not an area of tremendous concern in MS-related difficulty. The most common bowel problem is constipation and, when looked at carefully, it is often the patient's expectations that are the problem. It is healthy—and normal—to have a movement once every three or four days. Many people create bowel troubles themselves by overdiagnosing and overtreating what they think is constipation. With overuse of laxatives and enemas, the rectum gets overstretched and loses tone. So it's important first to rule out "nonproblems."

When constipation does exist in MS, it is usually the result of inactivity because the patient is not able to exercise or walk as much as before. This decreases bowel stimulation. Here, an increase in physical activity often solves the problem. Other commonsense measures include use of medication and change in diet. Fiber, oil, and abundant fluids are all vital to regularity.

Most constipation can be prevented before it occurs by getting the proper amount of exercise and eating a good diet that includes bran, fruits, vegetables, and a good intake of fluids. If the person has some limitations in walking, then proper exercise should include a stationary bike or swimming. There is always some way for the MS patient to exercise.

Once the patient is educated in the range of normal regularity, and it is determined that constipation does exist, treatment can begin. The patient should first set aside adequate time in the bathroom. Twenty or thirty minutes after breakfast or morning coffee is probably the most opportune time because a bowel reflex occurs naturally upon filling the stomach. If twenty or thirty minutes is difficult to fit into your schedule, get up a half-hour earlier.

If simple measures are not enough, then medications which provide bulk, such as Metamucil, and medications that provide lubrication, such as Ex-Lax and other laxatives, can be tried. However, laxatives, along with enemas, should always be a last resort. When constipation is severe, the patient should see a gastroenterologist for retraining of the bowels and evaluation of bad habits that may have accumulated. Fecal impactions and blockage of the rectum, which can be self-diagnosed with the fingers, require immediate attention.

Incontinence, or the loss of bowel control, is extremely rare for the MS patient. When it does occur, it is often due to fecal impaction rather than permanent loss of rectal control. When incontinence does occur, medication to inhibit bladder spasms may work, and bowel retraining, including biofeedback, may be effective. But this situation is so rare that it should not be one of the worries of the MS patient.

Sexual Dysfunction

Sexual dysfunction in MS may be either physical or psychological. Sometimes it's difficult for the neurologist to separate the two. But the patient should be able to tell if the problem is lack of desire, caused by depression or anxiety, or decreased ability to have an erection or orgasm.

It's very normal for everyone, with or without MS, occasionally to have sexual difficulty. If a person becomes anxious, the situation may be prolonged. Untreated anxiety about sexual function can even create a permanent problem that sadly, the patient believes is an effect of MS. This type of problem is evident in the man who has trouble completing intercourse or has a weak erection or trouble maintaining an erection, although he can experience a good erection in his sleep or on waking in the morning. This is evidence that the physical function is there and that an emotional disturbance is interfering. With women, discerning sexual dysfunction from an emotional problem is more difficult. The woman with MS-related orgasmic difficulty may have numbness of the genital area.

In MS, true physical sexual dysfunction is almost always associated with weakness or spasticity of the legs or bladder-control problems. Often treatment of these problems will clear up the sexual problem, so it's important to examine each to see exactly where the difficulty lies.

Rarely, the genital area becomes supersensitive to touch or

a burning sensation occurs. This can be relieved by spraying the area with ethyl chloride or applying anesthetic lotion or ointment. Medications for numbness and tingling may also work.

If sexual dysfunction is a persistent problem of a physical origin, then imaginative measures should be taken to make the sex act pleasurable in spite of this.

Popular medications for alleviating erectile dysfunction in men, such as Viagra, Levitra, and Cialis, may be successful whether the problem is physical or psychological.

Finally, communication and assertiveness in the bedroom will help a couple discover alternative means for enhancing the sexual experience. Using other parts of the body, along with imagination, creativity, and fantasy, will help change the approach to sex. Every person with MS should expect sexual pleasure and be able to find it no matter what the problem. If this proves to be difficult, sexual counseling can help couples overcome shyness and inhibitions.

Lack of Energy

With MS it is very common to recover completely from an attack except for the fatigue that lingers for months afterwards. Frequently, the patient is completely normal for years, except for what is probably the most common residual symptom—lack of energy.

Traditionally, coffee and tea are good stimulants. And many patients believe that daily shots of vitamin B_{12} give them a boost. This has never been proved scientifically, only anecdotally from patients. Brewer's yeast, in a dosage of up to thirty tablets a day, is a simpler step to gain more energy.

The antiviral flu medication, amantadine (Symmetrel), is sometimes effective in relieving fatigue in people with

MS. Side effects might include dry mouth, dizziness, trouble concentrating, and irritability. Prozac, a popular drug for treatment of depression, can also help to alleviate MS-related fatigue.

When fatigue is the patient's main problem, everything that could possibly affect energy must be looked at. Is the person refusing to use a walking stick for long distances? Is depression the cause of fatigue? Is urinary frequency causing interruption of sleep? Is the daily routine efficient?

Reorganizing daily activities can often have a dramatic effect on the patient's energy. Very often the person can accomplish more in the beginning of the day and less in the afternoon. If this is the case, as many chores and errands as possible should be gotten out of the way early and a rest break should be taken later on. Also, sit down at every opportunity. Standing eats up valuable energy that you would rather store. Can you trade certain taxing chores with others in the household? Are you trying too hard to prove to yourself and everyone else that you can do everything? Let the kids and your friends help out. If you didn't have MS, you would probably insist, so don't become a martyr now.

If necessary, keep a log for one week and write down what you do throughout each day. Put a notation at the points when you get tired. Look at it as if it were a battle plan, and restructure your schedule where needed. Your fatigue is real, but if you take the offensive, you can reduce it greatly.

Cognitive Impairment

Problems with attention, information processing, memory, planning, or problem solving can affect 50 to 65 percent of people with MS. It is believed the loss of myelin, the insulating material around nerve fibers, can interrupt the transportation of memories to storage areas in the brain.

MS has the potential to affect personality, emotions, and intellect through the loss of myelin, damage to the fibers, or loss of brain tissue. While mild problems are common (40 percent of people with MS have mild dysfunction), severe damage to these brain functions is rare. Only 5 to 10 percent of people with MS will have moderate to severe impairment. There is no correlation between physical disability and cognitive deficits, according to several studies. Fatigue and cognitive impairment do show a correlation in some studies. Medications, sleeplessness, nutrition, menopause, and depression can also add to cognitive problems and should be assessed as well.

While research shows nine out of ten people with MS are free of severe intellectual problems, cognitive impairment is one of the major reasons cited for unemployment among people with MS. So it's important to screen, assess, and manage. Many studies have shown that lesion volume is correlated with cognitive impairment, especially in the cerebral area. Stronger correlations are shown with brain atrophy as opposed to extent of lesions. A goal for researchers should be to identify at-risk patients. Since the consequences of intellectual impairment can be great, identification and intervention are critical. Often the patient is reluctant, even unaware. Family reports may be helpful.

Keeping employment, remaining independent, and improving function are realistic goals. There are many memory exercises and tricks used by experts. "Repeat and Verify" helps many with names. "See it, Say it, Hear It, Write it, Do It," is another method to help memory.

Use a daily planner and calendar—just one—and learn to rely on it. Use an alarm watch or electronic organizer with reminders. Be organized, and simplify your lists. Eliminate distractions. Although we live in a multitasking world, the person fighting memory problems should turn off the TV or radio when speaking with someone in person or on the phone. You can restore many functions and compensate for those still impaired.

EMOTIONAL LABILITY AND DEPRESSION

Although rare, some patients with brain stem attacks may have emotional lability—sudden outbursts of inappropriate laughing or crying. The patient may cry without control at a sentimental episode on TV or laugh when the knee reflex is tapped. This may be in isolation or associated with speech difficulty. Emotional lability is treatable with two different medications—tranquilizers such as Valium or antidepressants such as Elavil. A good compromise is Triavil, a tranquilizer and antidepressant. Sometimes euphoria, a feeling of well-being not justified by circumstances, is present. It is rarely noticed when mild. In more severe cases, mood-altering medication may be indicated.

Depression is a much more common problem. We have only recently learned that 50 to 60 percent of people with MS will experience a major depressive incident, much higher risk than the 17 percent of the general population. It is often difficult to discern whether it's a direct result of the pathology of MS or an emotional reaction to the MS diagnosis and the subsequent difficulty of coping. But much of it is now believed to be organic to the disease process.

Depression can also be a side effect of medication. Amantadine, for instance, lists depression as one of its more rare side effects, but it can happen. Research has failed to show a strong link between depression and interferon treatment, but beta-interferon is known to decrease levels of serotonin in the brain, which is linked to depression.

Regardless of the cause, major depression does affect people with MS at some point in their lives. It is not a passing mood, not the "blues" that everyone experiences. A major episode, according to the American Psychiatric Association, has five or more of the following symptoms for at least two weeks:

- Feeling sad or empty or being irritable or tearful most of the day
- Loss of interest or pleasure in most activities
- Significant weight loss or gain or dramatic change in appetite
- Sleeping too much or not at all
- Physical restlessness or slowed movement observed by others
- Ongoing fatigue or loss of energy
- Feeling worthless or guilty without appropriate cause
- Diminished ability to concentrate or make decisions
- Recurrent thoughts of death or suicide, or planning suicide

One or both of the first two symptoms are always present in a major depressive episode. Once depression is acknowledged, it should be treated immediately.

There are many antidepressants on the market that restore the brain's normal chemical balance by slowing the removal of certain chemicals called neurotransmitters. Serotonin and norepinephrine are the two chemicals antidepressants target. Most medications work gradually and after about six weeks the doctor can evaluate the dose and decide to add another medication or prescribe a different drug. It is trial and error and, needless to say, a challenge to tailor the right treatment to each patient.

Older antidepressants such as amitriptyline (Elavil),

imipramine hydrochloride (Tofranil), doxepin (Sinequan, Adapin), alprazolam (Xanax), trazodone hydrochloride (Desyrel), and amitriptyline with chlordiazepoxide (Limbitrol) are effective.

But a newer group of antidepressants known as SSRIs are gaining in popularity because they tend to have fewer side effects. The SSRIs, selective serotonin reuptake inhibitors, include fluoxetine (Prozac), sertraline (Zoloft), fluvoxamine (Luvox), paroxetine (Paxil), escitalopram oxalate (Lexapro), and citalopram (Celexa). And in the late 1990s, a new group of drugs, SSRNIs, were developed to target both serotonin and norepinephrine levels. Popular SSRNIs include duloxetine (Cymbalta), venlafaxine (Effexor), and nefazodone (Serzone).

Additional newcomers, unrelated to the other antidepressants, include bupropion (Wellbutrin) and mirtazapine (Remeron).

The most common side effects of the newer drugs include sexual problems, headache, insomnia, jittery feelings, and weight loss or gain. As people with MS learn all too quickly, few medications are without side effects. Again, each patient must weigh the benefit against the side effects. For some, talk therapy is a better course. For many, antidepressants can work like a miracle.

One final thought: Increasing levels of disability do not have to equal depression. A study once compared the "happiness set point" of people who were paralyzed in accidents. Trained professionals observed that within eighteen months of their life traumas, those paralyzed had returned to their previous levels of happiness. Another study looked at the happiness levels of new lottery winners. Within eighteen months of their momentary life "highs," the lottery winners settled back into their original happiness set points as well. If they were happy before, they were happy after. If they were miserable before, they weren't any different after. The key to it all: a long-range coping strategy.

Alternative Therapies and Therapeutic Claims

One study in 1997 revealed that 40 percent of people with MS had tried alternative therapies, half in combination with prescription medicine. As many as 60 percent of that group did not discuss this with their doctors. The list of tried-and-failed treatments is long, and not meant to be discouraging. In fact, this process of elimination has led investigators closer to the real answers. The "alternative" therapies that have stood the test of time, such as steroid treatment, have become the conventional therapies.

Today, with such breakthroughs in disease-modifying drugs, people with MS need to turn to alternative therapies less and less. However, some people with symptoms or progression that has not been helped with anything traditional medicine has had to offer believe in the philosophy of "try anything" for relief and well-being. After all, the popular heart disease treatment, digitalis, begins with a plant, *Digitalis lanata*. A group of active compounds are extracted primarily from the leaves of the second year's growth, and in pure form are referred to by brand names such as Lanoxin or Purgoxin. You can't try a home remedy here. The entire plant—leaves, seed, roots—is poisonous. Just a nibble is enough to cause death, earning it the nicknames "Dead Man's Bells" and "Witches' Gloves." In pharmaceutical form, however, it strengthens heart muscles and controls irregular and often fast heart beats.

So why is there so much skepticism that other plants don't offer other medical benefits? It is primarily because there are few controlled studies of safety and effectiveness, let alone experiments with amounts and delivery systems. Many herbs are known to have potent properties. Take the herb thyme, that you probably have on your spice shelf. Online today, you can read a fact sheet from the U.S. Environmental Protection Agency approving thyme for use as a pesticide to control aphids on plants in ponds, fountains, and other aquatic sites.

Thyme has a long history of use in natural medicine. During the Middle Ages, thyme was grown in monastery gardens in southern France and in Spain and Italy for use as a cough remedy, digestive aid, and treatment for intestinal parasites. Thyme's most active ingredient, thymol, is used in such over-the-counter products as Listerine mouthwash and Vicks VapoRub because of its well-known antibacterial and antifungal properties. Thymol apparently also has a therapeutic effect on the lungs. Ingesting or inhaling the oil helps to loosen phlegm and relax the muscles in the respiratory tract.

In Germany, concoctions of thyme are frequently prescribed for coughs, including those resulting from whooping cough, bronchitis, and emphysema. In the United States, thyme extract was included in a popular cough syrup that is no longer on the market. In addition, thyme has also been used against athlete's foot. Its primary ingredients are flavonoids (apigenin, luteolin, eriodicytol), tannins, bitter compounds, resin, saponin, and volatile oils (thymol, methylchavicol, cineole, and borneol). Thymol is the most valuable for medicinal purposes (but carvacrol, an isomeric phenol, is present in some oils).

So what does this have to do with MS? Perhaps nothing, but recent studies show that thymol interacts with GABA receptors, which are present on most nerve cells in the brain. These bind with benzodiazepines (Valium), barbiturates, and alcohol, and an amino acid called GABA (gamma-aminobutryic acid). GABA is actually classified as a neurotransmitter, which means it helps nerve impulses cross the synapses (gaps) and communicate better.

When GABA is in the normal range in the brain, we are not overly excitable or anxious. At the same time, we have appropriate reactions to situations in our environment. GABA is also the communication speed controller, making sure all brain communications are operating at the right speed and with the correct intensity. With too little GABA in the brain, the communication becomes out of control, overstimulated, and chemically unstable. Too much GABA and we are overly relaxed and sedated, often to the point that normal reactions are impaired. Researchers at the City of Hope in Duarte, CA, were the first to report that a GABA gene is associated with MS. But no one knows yet what this means.

Thyme is not the only herb or supplement which interacts with GABA receptors. Kava kava, valerian, St. John's wort, vitamin B_6, manganese, taurine, and lysine also are believed to have involvement as well. But what do you take and when? Are there other dangers? Perhaps. Back to thyme: Casual browsing of health food sites found this warning: "Due to immune stimulating properties, Thyme Essential Oil should not be used topically on people who have an autoimmune disease."

Whether they're used to season food, taken as supplements, even used for baths or massages, herbs can have powerful effects on the body. The National Institutes of Health recently reported that three adolescent boys developed breasts after bathing in lavender bath products, something which stimulated an odd hormonal reaction. The vast majority of herbs, however, are safe for consumption or use in essential oils, creams, and fragrances. Some problems are due to inconsistent strengths and/or purity, untested dose recommendations, side effects, and, most serious of all, known and unknown drug-herb interactions. Researchers cannot possibly test all combinations. Yet Americans have spoken with their pocketbooks. Last year alone, they spent $27 billion for products, classes, and books. So we advise that if you use herbs, follow simple but sensible guidelines in self-treatment:

- Do talk to your doctor and review any possible drug interactions.
- Use only herbs recommended in respected herb books.
- Avoid products with claims of "wonder treatments."
- Immediately discontinue use if adverse reactions occur.
- Seek medical treatment for suspected adverse reactions.

So with all the caveats above, and with hope that more doctors will help guide their patients who want these options, here is a list of the more popular alternative treatments and what we know about the risks, the efficacy, and in some cases, the promise.

Categories of alternative treatments:

1. Treatments that increase blood flow
2. Treatments that decrease blood clotting
3. Treatments of chemical excess or deficiency
4. Treatments of the immune system
5. Miscellaneous treatments

Treatments that Increase Blood Flow

Because MS lesions begin around small blood vessels, researchers once believed that spasms or blockages at these sites might be the cause of the disease. Thus, attempts were made to improve blood flow to the brain, prevent blockage, and therefore prevent future attacks.

The heat box, fever therapies, and blood vessel dilators, called vasodilators, work on the principle of increasing blood flow or decreasing viscosity. Hydergine, amyl nitrite, aminophylline, papaverine, alcohol, diphenhydramine, benzazoline hydrochloride, belladona, and tetraethylammonium are among the many vasodilator drugs tried unsuccessfully over the years in the treatment of MS.

In MS, histamine therapy was widespread for about fifteen years. Histamine is a chemical found in the body that alters the size of the blood vessels. Today we are more familiar with its effective use in treatment of allergies. The first MS trial, in 1944, was heralded as a success. Even though it was uncontrolled, doctors reported recovery in 75 percent of acute attacks and improvement in 46 percent of chronic cases. Later, however, a controlled test showed no improvements.

Circulation stimulants that raise blood pressure were also tested in the treatment of MS. The list of stimulants includes caffeine, alcohol, ephedrine, adrenocortical extract, desoxycorticosterone acetate (DOCA) and neostigmine. In all, forty cases were studied and some appeared to have good results, but no exact statistics were ever furnished.

Treatments that Decrease Blood Clotting

Heparin, an anticoagulant that decreases blood clotting, was first tried in 1959 in the treatment of acute MS attacks and chronic stages. But neither disease progression nor the attacks were reduced.

Clofibrate (Atromid-S), an agent that reduces fat and cholesterol in the blood, was tried in a twenty-month controlled study of MS patients. Results from the experimental group were, for the most part, the same as from the control group.

In 1947 a neurologist reported that another anticoagulant, dicumarol, helped reduce MS attacks. But another study five years later showed no benefits from the treatment. Today dicumarol is considered ineffective and dangerous, as it is known to have caused fatal hemorrhages.

Treatments of Chemical Excess or Deficiency

Diets

Because epidemiology studies show varying MS incidence in different geographical locations and among different races, nutrition has been an area of great interest in MS research for many years. Diet treatments follow four theories—that MS is caused by (1) a deficiency in or excess of a food, (2) a toxic effect of a food, (3) an allergic reaction to a food, or (4) the ingestion of the "MS agent." Some diet treatments over the years have been proved ineffective, while others have not been proved or disproved but rather have failed to stand the test of time. In all fairness, the testing of diets has always been difficult. Outside a controlled hospital environment, it is estimated that only one-third of those tested will adhere strictly to a prescribed diet. With that in mind, here are the best-known diets people with MS are likely to come across.

Low-Fat Diet: The first serious modern claim for an "MS diet" was made in 1950, when Dr. Roy Swank of Oregon suggested that in geographical locations around the world with higher MS populations, the intake of fat in the diet is greater. Supporting this theory was the belief that fat particles in the blood, or possibly blockage in blood vessels, could cause myelin damage. None of this, however, could explain why white South Africans had a high-fat diet and low MS incidence. Ultimately, a study of a large group of MS patients followed for seventeen years proved the low-fat diet had no effect on the course of the disease. A lower death rate, along with reduction in frequency of attacks, was reported, however. The low-fat diet, of course, is a healthy diet in general and will improve general health by keeping weight down, lowering blood pressure, and preventing arteriosclerosis. These factors are more likely to have influenced the good test results. The low-fat diet is actually the favorite diet of the American Heart Association, and one I recommend, but not necessarily as a treatment for MS.

Low-Gluten Diet: This diet, first introduced in Melbourne, Australia, by Dr. R. Shatin, was based on the analysis that geographical locations with high MS incidence have higher consumption of wheat and rye products, or of gluten. Shatin advocated a balanced diet that substituted rice and corn for wheat and rye products, as well as lowered intake of coffee, alcohol, and carbohydrates. Both controlled and uncontrolled studies showed this diet was ineffective and difficult to stay on. Today, the low-gluten diet is only recommended for those with wheat or rye allergies.

The MacDougall Diet: The MacDougall Diet, developed by Roger MacDougall, a writer and dramatist, is a combination of low-fat and gluten-free diets. Professor MacDougall claimed his diet caused his own MS symptoms to disappear, but broader scientific evidence of this has yet to be shown.

Allergen-free Diet: This diet, still used by some today, is based on the theory that MS lesions might actually be the result of the body's own allergic reaction to something in the environment. So, to prevent future attacks, the patient eliminates from the diet those substances to which he or she is allergic. A few clinics promise a new approach to managing MS with this treatment, but no scientific studies have proved or disproved its effectiveness.

The Evers Diet: Developed by a German physician, Dr. Joseph Evers, this diet treatment is based on the theory that

MS, like many other illnesses, is caused by eating unnatural foods. The Evers diet, therefore, consists of all raw, natural foods, plus wheat germ. Salt, sugar, and condiments are forbidden, as are salads, asparagus, and cauliflower. Only natural wines and brandies are permitted. No scientific evidence of the effectiveness of the Evers diet has ever been shown, though before his death in 1977, he treated more than 15,000 patients.

In conclusion, diets are all right as long as the MS patient isn't weakened to the point of becoming susceptible to infection. Diet does play a part in the management of MS, but only in keeping weight at a normal level. Intense crash diets are not recommended for anyone; they can lead to potassium deficiency and other problems.

Nutritional Supplements

Vitamins: Since the 1920s the notion that MS is the result of an unidentified vitamin deficiency has been around, and supplements, both in liquid and capsule form, have been advocated. Many vitamin therapies have been tested, including ascorbic acid (vitamin C), thiamine (B_1), vitamin B_{12}, niacin, vitamin E, and liver therapy. Vitamins A, D, E, and K have also been combined with thiamine, niacin, and ammonium chloride. Improvements have been reported as zero percent in some studies, 100 percent in others. Unfortunately, most test results are of an anecdotal nature without controlled scientific evaluation.

Megavitamins: Megavitamin therapy—the taking of massive doses of nutritional supplements that exceed one thousand times the minimum daily required dose—has been touted, but also without reliable scientific evidence. Most researchers consider megavitamins to be "an expensive placebo." All patients should make sure they get the minimum daily requirements as a general rule. But those taking extra vitamins should be aware that too much vitamin A and D are dangerously toxic. Too much vitamin B_6 can result in numbness, loss of balance, and weakness *apart* from MS symptoms.

Antioxidants: Free radicals are chemicals that can damage cells in a process called oxidative damage. Some studies have shown that this process may be involved in MS. Studies of EAE, the animal model of MS, have shown antioxidants can decrease the severity of the disease. Common antioxidants include vitamins A, C, and E, and selenium. Less common compounds include alpha-lipoic acid, uric acid, inosine, coenzyme Q10 (CoQ10), grape seed extract, pycnogenol, and oligomeric proanthocyanidins (OPCs). Recent studies have shown that alpha-lipoic and uric acids are effective therapies with EAE. And clinical studies on people with MS are now underway testing alpha-lipoic acid and ionosine, a compound that is converted to uric acid. One risk, in theory, is that antioxidants may stimulate T cells, and potentially aggravate the disease. More studies are needed.

Minerals: Since the 1880s when Charcot tested the use of zinc phosphates, minerals have been used in therapies for MS. Today essential minerals are combined with vitamin supplements. Zinc, still in use today, does activate T cells in the immune system, which can cause worsening of the disease. High zinc levels are also associated with low blood levels of copper and an MS-like condition called copper-deficiency myelopathy and neurological symptoms that are similar to MS.

Recently, one researcher reported a manganese deficiency in MS patients and advocated an increase in the consumption of buckwheat pancakes, a food rich in manganese. It certainly is not harmful, but there is no proof that adding manganese to the diet helps prevent MS attacks or slow worsening.

Polyunsaturated Fatty Acids: Supplementing the diet with polyunsaturated fatty acids (PUFA) such as safflower oil, sunflower seed oil, evening primrose oil, or linoleic acid has been investigated, rejected as a therapy, and investigated again. Many of my own patients have tried these supplements, some for as long as twenty years, without any success. Three scientifically controlled studies on large MS groups shows some slightly favorable effects that were first discounted by the National MS Society and then reconsidered. One study showed that the PUFA group had a slight reduction in frequency of attacks, and another study showed a reduction in severity of attacks. PUFA did not, however, show any overall effect on the progression of the disease. It has been suggested that some sources of PUFA, such as sunflower seed oil, are more beneficial than others, such as evening primrose oil. Although it seems unlikely that this is a cure, more studies are needed since such factors as the length of the study, the amount of PUFA, and the source of PUFA have varied.

PUFAs are commonly known now as omega-3 and omega-6 fatty acids. Omega-3 is found in relatively high levels in fatty fish such as salmon, Atlantic herring, Atlantic mackerel, bluefin tuna, and sardines. Dietary supplements include fish oil, cod liver oil, flaxseed oil, canola oil, and walnut oil. A small study evaluated omega-3 supplements (fish oil) taken with interferons or glatiramer acetate. The study showed a decrease in relapse rate and improved physical and emotional functioning. Omega-6 supplements include sunflower seed oil, evening primrose oil, flaxseed oil, borage seed oil, black currant seed oil, and spirulina (blue-green algae.) Some of these supplements have provoked seizures on rare occasion. Some have blood-thinning effects. Some can cause a rise in triglyceride levels. Borage seed oil may be toxic to the liver. And spirulina supplements may contain bacteria and other contaminants. Those cautions aside, PUFAs have shown enough encouraging results over the years to warrant further clinical studies.

Gingko biloba, a popular supplement that comes from

the leaf of the gingko biloba tree, is best known for its anti-inflammatory and antioxidant effects. It can improve memory and cognitive function in people with Alzheimer's disease, and studies are currently underway to see if it has similiar benefits for people with MS. So far, it has not shown to be effective in treating MS attacks. Further studies are needed to see if it can prevent attacks or slow the course of MS. The herb may cause dizziness, rashes, headache, and gastrointestinal distress and has a blood-thinning effect. In rare cases it may provoke seizures.

Kava kava is from the root of the kava plant and was first used in Europe in the nineteenth century to treat venereal disease. Today it is used for anxiety. The plant compounds, called kavalactones, interact with GABA receptors. Several clinical trials show kava kava is effective for mild anxiety, but not for more severe anxiety. Kava intensifies the effects of alcohol, benzodiazepines, and other psychoactive drugs. Kava used with alprazolam has resulted in a coma. Long-term use has caused yellow skin discoloration. But the most serious side effect has been fifty reports of liver toxicity in the past few years, some of which led to death or the need for a transplant, leading to the banning of kava in several countries.

Padma 28: In the late nineteenth century, two Russian doctors developed a mixture of more than twenty herbs thought to suppress the immune system and produce antioxidant effects. This formulation had also been carried by Tibetan Buddhists, philosophers, and doctors in the eighteenth century to the West, finally arriving in Switzerland in the 1960s. One formula was preserved by Karl Lutz, and is manufactured commercially today by a Swiss company PADMA AG, with each tablet containing the following ingredients:

- Allspice 25mg
- Bengal Quince 20mg

- Cardamom 30mg
- Cloves 12mg
- Columbine 15mg
- Gingerlily 10mg
- Heartleaved Sida 10mg
- Iceland Moss 40mg
- KnotGrass 15mg
- Licorice 15mg
- Margosa 35mg
- Marigold 5mg
- Myrobalan 30mg
- Potentilla Golden Herb 15mg
- Red Sandalwood 30mg
- Ribwort 15mg
- Saussuria 40mg
- Valerian 10mg
- Wild Lettuce 6mg
- Calcium Sulphate 20mg
- Camphor 4mg
- Silicon Dioxide 12mg
- Sorbitol 73mg

There has been limited research, although one clinical study of a hundred people with MS showed those who took the mixture had a less severe disease course (*Phytotherapy Research* 1992, 6:133–136). The 100 subjects suffering from a primary-progressive form of MS were randomly divided into two equal groups. Group 1 received Padma 28, two tablets three times a day, and group 2, the control group, was treated only for symptoms. After one year, 44 percent of the patients taking Padma 28 showed positive results including improvement of general condition, increase of muscle strength, and decrease or disappearance of disorders affecting sphincters. In 41 percent of patients with initially an abnormal tracing of visual evoked potentials, an improvement or normalization was achieved. Of patients who did not receive Padma 28, none felt better; moreover, 40 percent showed a deterioration. Tolerance of the drug was excellent. No side effects were reported. Better studies are needed.

St. John's wort is an herbal supplement that has been used as an antidepressant for more than 2,000 years. A 1996 analysis of twenty-three clinical studies involving 1,757 people showed St. John's wort alleviated mild to moderate depression, somehow changing the levels of some neurochemicals related to mood, such as serotonin and noradrenaline. It was not shown to help severe depression. Side effects include fatigue and sensitivity of the skin and nerves to sunlight. It may also affect dosage of oral contraceptives, heart medications, blood thinners, anticonvulsants, and other antidepressants.

Valerian, an herb, has been used as an insomnia remedy for more than 1,000 years. It has also been touted as a therapy for depression and spasticity. Several studies show it may be an effective treatment for insomnia, but further studies are needed. As it does have a sedating effect, caution must be taken when using other medications.

Chili peppers contain a substance called capsaicin, which is what makes them so spicy (the more capsaicin it contains, the spicier the pepper). Capsaicin is also an anti-inflammatory compound that, some say, helps with pain relief and many other ailments. This is basically anecdotal. Contrary to popular belief, chili peppers do not cause stomach ulcers. In fact, they help prevent them by killing bacteria you eat. They also contain vitamins C and A. Capsaicin is mostly in the chili pepper's seeds and white inner membrane, and is said to boost immunity and help fight off potential pathogens.

Clove: The active compound in cloves, eugenol, combines with other clove components to make this pungent spice highly antibacterial. It is also anti-inflammatory, and the compound has been studied for use in preventing:

- Toxicity from environmental pollutants
- Digestive tract cancers
- Joint inflammation

Because clove extracts are antibacterial and provide a mild anesthetic, they are used in the United States for dental procedures such as root canal therapy and temporary fillings. They are used in some sore throat sprays and mouthwashes. They are also an excellent source of traditional nutrients, including omega-3 fatty acids, dietary fiber, vitamin C and magnesium.

Garlic: Allicin, a compound found in garlic (and the one that gives it its odor), is believed to have powerful antibacterial and antiviral properties. When combined with the vitamin C in garlic, this compound can kill harmful microbes and fight diseases including cold and flu, stomach viruses, and Candida yeast. Claims have also been made that it can fight tuberculosis and botulism, although anyone would certainly go to a hosptial for treatments of those serious conditions. Garlic is also known to lower blood pressure, insulin requirements for those with diabetes, and triglycerides. In animals, allicin has been shown to help prevent weight gain. A study published in the December 2003 issue of the *American Journal of Hypertension* found that rats' weights remained stable or decreased slightly when allicin was given along with a sugar-rich diet, while other rats' weights increased.

Mustard Seed: Researchers from the University of Manitoba in Winnipeg, Canada, found that the antimicrobial properties of mustard seed are so strong that, when added to hamburger meat, it could kill E. coli bacteria. The compound responsible for this is allyl isothiocyanate. The U.S. Department of Agriculture reported that this compound can also kill listeria, Staphylococcus aureus, and other food-borne pathogens. The prepared mustard typically consumed in the United States does not contain allyl isothiocyanate.

Sage is believed to be an anti-inflammatory, antioxidant, and powerful antimicrobial, and is known to kill Candida albicans and salmonella. Sage leaf extract is also known to kill the microbe that causes gingivitis. Sage may also be good for your brain. A study in the June 2003 *Pharmacological Biochemical Behavior* found that people given sage essential oil extracts had significantly improved recall abilities compared to those given a placebo.

Rosemary: Traditionally, rosemary has been used by herbalists to relieve muscle pain and spasm, stimulate hair growth, and support the circulatory and nervous systems. It is also believed to affect the menstrual cycle, act as an abortifacient (inducing miscarriage), relieve menstrual cramps, increase urine flow, and reduce kidney pain (for example, from kidney stones).

Rosemary has been regarded by some as a memory enhancer. That belief can be traced back to ancient Greece, where students would put sprigs of rosemary in their hair while studying. It has also been used to treat alopecia, a disease (of unknown origin) causing significant hair loss, usually in patches. In one study of eighty-six people with alopecia, those who massaged their scalps with rosemary and other essential oils (including lavender, thyme, and cedarwood) every day for seven months experienced significant hair regrowth compared to those who massaged their scalps without the essential oils. It is not entirely clear from this study whether rosemary (or a combination of rosemary and the other essential oils) was responsible for the beneficial effects.

In one laboratory study, rosemary extract increased the

effectiveness of doxorubicin in treating human breast cancer cells. Further studies on humans are needed, but meanwhile, those taking doxorubicin should consult their doctors if taking rosemary. Both laboratory and animal studies suggest that rosemary's antioxidant properties may have activity against colon, breast, stomach, lung, and skin cancer cells. Much more research in this area must be conducted before conclusions can be drawn about the value of rosemary. For treatment of multiple sclerosis, the National Multiple Sclerosis Society says on its Web site that rosemary essential oil is "good for MS," adding "essential oils are able to penetrate the skin and enter the bloodstream. Some essential oils have anti-inflammatory properties; others bring about a feeling of relaxation; others are stimulating. . . ." They believe rosemary is a neuromuscular relaxant.

Aloe Vera: Aloe vera juice, high in vitamins, amino acids, and minerals, can be a healthy food supplement, but its value in the treatment of MS has not been substantiated. Some MS patients claim to have recovered from acute attacks after taking the juice, but this is most likely due to the natural course of the attack and remission. There is no scientific data that show aloe vera to be an effective treatment for MS.

Adenosine-5-Monophosphate: Also known as C_3A_5MP, this is a chemical found normally in the nerves and muscles. In the 1950s a doctor who had MS self-administered this chemical, believing that MS might be caused by a deficiency of it. He claimed his MS improved and stayed better, but trials in many clinics failed to support his findings.

Cerebrosides: Cerebrosides, fatty acids found in beef spinal cord, were tested on MS patients for a period of a year and a half in scientifically controlled groups. The results showed this supplement to be ineffective.

Pancreatic Enzymes: In the 1950s and 1960s, Dr. Clinton Thienes of the Huntington Memorial Hospital MS Clinic in

Pasadena, California, believed that beef pancreas, injected into the muscle, had a therapeutic value in MS treatment. In some cases speech and spasticity improved to some degree, but the progressive cases showed no change. In all, this treatment is considered ineffective. It has also been tried in pill form, since repeated injections of large, foreign molecules can cause life-threatening reactions.

Chelation

Chelation treatment has legitimate uses in medicine today since it removes excess amounts of metal and minerals from the body. It is used effectively in heavy-metal poisoning, including lead, arsenic, and mercury. Unfortunately, chelation treatment is used inappropriately for arteriosclerosis and multiple sclerosis. There is no scientific basis for these treatments, and they are not recommended. Side effects include nausea, vomiting, and kidney damage.

Replacement of Dental Fillings

In the early 1980s, a few dentists claimed that MS was either caused by or aggravated by silver mercury used to fill cavities. The dentists advocated that this type of filling be replaced by either gold or plastic. In earlier literature a Swiss neurologist, Ernst Baasch, claimed a link between mercury toxicity and MS. Other reports suggested that a combination of gold and silver fillings with saliva causes neurological problems. The pure numbers of people with dental fillings versus those with MS make this theory very unlikely. Also, MS has been around much longer than modern dentistry. The replacement of fillings as a treatment for

MS also remains highly suspicious on the basis that those who advocate it make a great profit from it.

AROMATHERAPY

The therapeutic use of essential oils has been around for thousands of years. For treatment of multiple sclerosis, the NMMS recommends essential oils of juniper as well as rosemary. Essential oils can be used for a soothing massage, an inhalant, for use in a bath or fragrance in a room. Essential oils should be diluted . . . a few drops in the bath or a bowl of water in the room to inhale. They must also be diluted before use directly on the skin. In addition to rosemary, the NMMS suggests black pepper oil for constipation; juniper for water retention; chamomile for sleep disturbances; and green apple fragrance to reduce headaches. Aromatherapy has never before been scientifically tested, but it is currently undergoing trials at NHS hospitals to see if it reduces pain and anxiety and if it can treat infections.

Also widely marketed, but not mentioned by the NMSS, is lavender, which consists of essential oils with over 100 compounds. It is commonly used to reduce tension, restlessness, depression, and insomnia. Lavender has been shown to cause sedative effects in rats. Caution is suggested when using alcohol or other sedative drugs. Adverse reactions include constipation, skin irritation, headache, and nausea. It is considered poisonous if swallowed.

Lemon balm is a member of the mint family that has been used to relieve anxiety and insomnia. As an inhalant, it is used for Alzheimer's disease. As aromatherapy it is well tolerated. Ingested, it can cause nausea, vomiting, dizziness, and stomach pain.

Skullcap is used for its calming effect on the body, to relieve insomnia, and to lessen the symptoms of alcohol withdrawal. Adverse reactions include liver toxicity and, in overdose, seizures or stupor. It may interact with and cause an altered effect on serum immunoglobins.

Treatments to Prevent Infection

Today, as mentioned earlier, we can successfully treat attacks that are triggered by infection. Beyond that, many attempts have been made to find and prevent the action of an infectious agent that may be the cause of MS itself. If the "MS agent" is well hidden in the brain or spinal cord, its detection will be difficult. In the 1950s and 1960s, scientists attempted to treat MS with antibiotics. Before the widespread availability of penicillin after 1944, drugs used for syphilis were used to treat MS. More recently an antiviral agent, arabinoside-A, that is effective against the herpes virus was tested for MS. But because of its toxic effect on the kidneys it is not recommended.

Even though anti-infective treatments have failed in the past, they may still be the hope for MS treatments in the future. Today anti-infective agents, particularly antiviral agents, are being tried at some of the best research clinics in the world. Since there is strong evidence that MS may be caused by a "slow virus," or a common viral infection in childhood, these treatments remain under aggressive investigation.

Amantadine

Amantadine (Symmetrel) has been shown to have some effect in preventing the flu, which can prevent flu-related MS attacks. Amantadine has also been proposed as a treatment to prevent all MS attacks or slow worsening. However, a thirty-six-month double-blind study showed it to be of no value in actually altering the course of MS. More recently it has also been suggested that amantadine may help the chronic fatigue associated with MS. The results have been mixed, and we believe it may be worth trying.

Cranberry Juice

For decades, cranberry juice has been used to prevent urinary tract infections. Two chemicals in cranberry juice, fructose and proanthocyanidin, kill some bacteria and help prevent them from adhering to the urinary tract wall. Limited studies show cranberry juice does help prevent UTIs in people with normal bladder function, but is not effective with people who have abnormal bladder function. Remember, it can be effective for *prevention.* If you have a known UTI, you must use prescription medication.

Yogurt Products/Probiotics

Progurt is a yogurt product from Australia, newly available in the United States, that makes the following big claim online:

> *Progurt has improved the quality of life of sufferers of Multiple Sclerosis. Progurt has been known to help long term sufferers of MS as well as those recently diagnosed. You may attain positive results within hours or days depending upon the severity of your condition. Progurt may eliminate or lessen the severity of the following symptoms of Multiple Sclerosis:*
>
> - *bowel and bladder dysfunction*
> - *cognitive function, including problems with memory, attention, and problem-solving*
> - *balance, dizziness, and vertigo*
> - *emotional problems and/or depression*
> - *fatigue (also called MS lassitude)*
> - *difficulty in walking and coordination problems*

- *numbness or "pins and needles"*
- *tremors*
- *vision problems*
- *hearing loss*
- *headache*
- *speech and swallowing disorders*
- *seizures*
- *itching*
- *spasticity*

They continue: "People crippled with multiple sclerosis have become more mobile; diabetics have experienced improvement in circulation and general well being. We stress that Progurt is a health food, not a medicine. . . . But the fact is that it has certain effects on the metabolism which can directly affect many health outcomes."

It is true that yogurt can give people a sense of well-being. And for many people taking MS medications that may be harsh on the intestinal tract, eating yogurt, with all its natural bacteria, is often recommended. But to date, we have not found any studies that show yogurt changes the course of MS or alleviates symptoms. There is certainly a growing interest in *probiotics*, foods and dietary supplements that contain trillions of helpful bacteria normally found in the body. These bacteria may assist with digestion and help protect the body against harmful bacteria. They are found not only in Australia's Progurt, but also in newer American products such as some store-bought yogurts and "Kombucha" teas.

Dr. Michael Picca, a gastroenterologist at the Mayo Clinic reports, "One study in Sweden found that a group of employees who were given probiotics missed less work due to illness than did employees who were not given probiotics. Other studies have found probiotics to be helpful in managing the signs and symptoms of irritable bowel syndrome

(IBS)." But he notes that research is just beginning. Probiotic bacteria may turn out to support the immune systems of elderly people or those with weakened immune systems. And it seems to have promise for treating bacterial vaginosis, diarrhea, foodborn pathogens, and some infections. But what if probiotics stimulate the riskier immune functions in people with MS? It is simply uncharted territory at this time.

Treatments of the Immune System

The most exciting area in MS therapy today is the immune system. The evidence for involvement of the immune system is overwhelming, and the laboratory tests for measuring abnormalities are very sophisticated. Researchers can now successfully test spinal fluid to see whether or not a specific treatment is affecting the immunological abnormality.

As early as 1927, the immune system was suspected of causing MS lesions. Today this theory remains one of the most aggressive areas of research as scientists explore various immune reactions that might be the culprits. Various treatments are based on exciting new immune system research uncovered in the past ten years.

The attempt to alter the course of the disease through the treatment of the immune system still remains the greatest hope for the future. The disease-modifying treatments using interferons and monocolonal antibodies, discussed in chapter 6, will become more and more effective. The use of cortisone drugs and ACTH has stood the test of time in treating the acute attack. Long-term steroid treatment is not recommended because it suppresses the immune system so indiscriminately that it leaves the patient with an increased susceptibility to infections, some life-threatening.

The list of possible treatments includes the latest strategies for using immunosuppressants, immune system modifiers, immune system desensitization, along with the latest information on promising new drugs, transfer factor, interferon, monoclonal antibodies, copolymer-1, desensitization to myelin basic protein, and plasmapheresis. In this chapter, the earliest attempts at immune therapy will be discussed.

Cellular Therapy

Almost fifty years ago a clinic in Switzerland pioneered a therapy for disease in which ground-up tissue from unborn animals was injected into patients. Those with heart trouble got ground-up heart tissue; for stomach trouble, ground-up stomach tissue. MS patients received injections of ground-up fetal brain. Although no studies were ever conducted and one death has been reported, a few doctors, including one in Santa Monica, California, still use this treatment. It should be considered ineffective and possibly dangerous.

Russian Vaccine

The Russian vaccine, prepared with rabies virus, is sold throughout Europe and South America to treat MS. Every once in a while, I see a patient who has gone to a clinic for this treatment. It has no value whatsoever. Other doctors have noted that it doesn't even prevent attacks during treatment. This vaccine may actually be an antirabies vaccine.

Echinacea

Echinacea is one of several dietary supplements said to stimulate the immune system. Sold as a cold and flu preventive for years, the latest studies showed it is not effective in either preventing or lessening the severity of such viruses. In laboratories, echinacea has activated T cells and macrophages, which could theoretically worsen MS. Therefore, it is not recommended. Also known to activate T cells are alfalfa, Asian and Siberian ginseng, astragalus, cat's claw, garlic, maitake mushrooms, mistletoe, shiitake mushrooms, stinging nettle, and melatonin.

Miscellaneous Treatments

Hyperbaric Oxygen (HBO)

The hyperbaric oxygen chamber has been in the news as pop star Michael Jackson's answer to the fountain of youth. He allegedly uses it to prevent aging. Originally used as an effective therapy for "the bends"—the aftereffect of too-rapid ascent from deep-sea diving—HBO replaces nitrogen bubbles in the blood with oxygen. Through the years HBO has also been effectively used in treatment of burns and gas gangrene. In the past few years, this device has been touted as beneficial in treatment of memory loss, mental deterioration, and Alzheimer's disease. Some slight improvements have been reported with that condition but without lasting benefits. Patients became slightly more alert while in the oxygen chamber and also experienced a feeling of euphoria.

HBO was investigated as a treatment for MS with the rationale that breathing oxygen under increased pressure in a specially constructed chamber would improve the conduction of signals through the central nervous system. At first it appeared that treatment had definite benefits. But later, in controlled studies around the world, results were disappointing. In a report published in June 1986 in *Neurology*, a group of experts tested eighty-two patients at the Tobermory Hyperbaric Facility in Canada. Forty-one patients received twenty consecutive daily treatments of 100 percent oxygen followed by seven booster treatments over the course of six months. Forty-one patients in the control group received 12.5 percent oxygen. The results showed no significant difference in their

Kurtzke disability scores, magnetic resonance imaging, or evoked potentials tests.

Cobra Venom

Cobra and other snake venoms are treatments in search of a disease. This strange therapy has been proposed for a variety of mystery illnesses such as lupus, herpes, muscular dystrophy, amyotrophic lateral sclerosis, and multiple sclerosis. The use of cobra venom has been traced back to a person who suffered neurological symptoms after being bitten by a snake. This led researchers to wonder if snake venom had other effects on the stimulation of the nervous system. Clinics popped up everywhere and some still exist, although it is widely accepted that cobra venom has no beneficial effect in MS or any other disease.

Bee Venom

Bee venom therapy has been traced back to ancient Greece and Egypt. Bees, held by a pair of tweezers, are placed on certain areas of the body, allowing the bee to sting as many as forty times, usually three treatments a week. Animal studies have shown BVT to be ineffective or actually linked to worsening of the disease process. But there are some clues in the research that warrant further investigation. It may be that the bee stings trigger the body to produce an anti-inflammatory response that not only helps quiet the bee sting, but any other inflammatory condition as well, such as MS or arthritis.

More recent studies show that some chemical components of bee venom can inhibit production of enzymes and proteins linked to inflammation. Also, apamin, another chemical compound found in bee venom, is now known to inhibit potassium channels, the mechanism at work with 4-AP, a more conventional therapy that has been shown to lessen MS symptoms, especially those that are heat-sensitive. It is occasionally recommended for treatment of visual symptoms, but any bee sting near the eye area can actually cause optic neuritis, not help it. Bee venom is a harsh treatment, never properly tested. Side effects, in rare cases, can even be life threatening such as anaphylactic shock resulting from an allergic reaction.

Eastern Relaxation Technique

Various forms of yoga, meditation, tai chi, massage, and visualization are all known to lessen stress in some cases, relieve pain, and certainly give people a better sense of wellbeing. We have found some yoga classes given for people with MS who prefer to remain seated. Massage is often helpful for those who need relief from stiffening muscles. Caution should be taken by those who take steroids as that treatment can lead to osteoporosis, which might leave the patient vulnerable to fractures during massage.

Acupuncture

Acupuncture is a treatment of traditional Chinese medicine (TCM) that involves sticking slender needles into key points in the body to, in theory, release *chi* energy. Although the mechanisms of acupuncture are not fully understood by Western or Eastern doctors, there is some evidence that acupuncture causes the release of peptides in the central nervous system, that modulates sensory information traveling from the body to the brain. It is commonly used as an alternative treatment for some of the symptoms of multiple sclerosis, especially pain and spasticity. Acupuncture is usually viewed with considerable skepticism by the medical profession, but some qualified doctors do recommend it, especially for the pain associated with facial neuralgias (primarily trigeminal neuralgia). Strong claims have also been made for the help acupuncture provides easing numbness and neck pain. It may be that acupuncture is helpful for certain MS-related symptoms but not others. There are no side effects. However, it is recommended that acupuncture be used only in addition to conventional medicine and in consultation with your physician. And finally, certain symptoms such as urinary symptoms or depression should not be treated by acupuncture alone.

Chiropractic Treatments

Back pain is a common problem for people with MS, exacerbated by weakened leg muscles. Chiropractic practice is recognized as an effective treatment for back pain and injury. The basic principle of chiropractic treatment is that spinal manipulation can help musculoskeletal problems such as back pain, as well as improving a person's general state of health.

Cannabis (Marijuana)

A few years ago, you couldn't miss the headline: "Cannabis has been proven, for the first time, to be an effective treatment for the symptoms of multiple sclerosis." Scientists from the Institute of Neurology at University College London had shown that a compound in cannabis could prevent muscle tremor and spasticity caused by the MS model—in mice. The mice were injected with the cannabinoid tetrahydrocannabinol (THC) as well as three synthetic compounds. One, methanandamide, was similar to a cannabinoid produced naturally in the body. All had a significant ability to reduce both tremor and spasticity. A synthetic compound called WIN55 proved the most effective against tremors.

Researcher Dr. David Baker described the great results of one synthetic compound with great enthusiasm: "The effect was really startling. It was a question of now you see the tremor, now you don't."

In November 2003, the long-awaited results on a large marijuana study of 630 people with MS was published, with mixed results. The patients taking cannabis pills and synthetic substitutes reported they felt great reduction of pain and muscle stiffness, but the improvements could not be detected by doctors. One study leader, Dr. John Zajicek of the University of Plymouth in England, said the research raises questions about what's more important: a doctor's measurements or the patient's perspective.

But the debate continues. And in January 2007, a British couple who supplied thousands of bars of chocolate laced with cannabis to ease the pain of multiple sclerosis wound up in court. While her supporters cheered her on, one doctor issued a warning about cannabis use, especially smoking it when you have MS. First, the risk of lung cancer among cannabis smokers is twenty times greater than for regular tobacco smokers, and about 400 times that of nonsmokers. In addition, it has been discovered that long-term cannabis smokers may suffer a dramatic and obvious form of premature brain atrophy (brain shrinkage). This has become apparent by brain-scan studies of the brains of habitual cannabis users.

"It seems therefore grossly inappropriate that we should treat one established form of brain damage, due to the MS, with a method which results in even more extensive, and permanent, brain damage, due to the cannabis. In comparison, the damage due to the MS may be considered largely repairable, as can be seen in those suffering an acute relapse, after which the recovery process will often restore 90 percent or more of the function lost. Even more long-term damage, due to established disease, may soon be repairable using current research projects including brain cell implants or drugs such as neuroimmunophylins," added Dr. M. R. Lawrence.

Dimethyl Sulfoxide (DMSO)

DMSO is a substance that, when applied to the skin, facilitates the absorption of medicinal compounds through the skin. While it has been valuable in arthritis treatments, its use in MS treatment has been based on one doctor's promotion. Without any controlled studies, this doctor, who wasn't even a neurologist and had no understanding of multiple sclerosis and its nature, treated several hundred patients with no success. DMSO is a perfect example of an MS treatment promoted for profit. It is clearly ineffective. Although it is not harmful, its application leaves the patient with a strong fishy odor.

Procaine (KH_3 or Gerovital)

This "magical" remedy is popular all over Europe. Procaine, or Novocain in oral form, is supposed to benefit many diseases from arthritis to cancer, Parkinson's disease, and arteriosclerosis. It is also supposed to prevent aging and sexual impotence or reverse these conditions. The most prominent promoter of this treatment is Dr. Anna Aslan of Bucharest, Romania. Her clinic draws people from all over the world, including statesmen and celebrities who should know better. KH_3 is not approved by the U.S. Food and Drug Administration (FDA), but it is believed that tablets are smuggled in from the West Indies and Mexico just the same. Although procaine is used effectively as a heart medicine, in local surgery, and in skin creams for local burns such as sunburn, there is no evidence it should be used for MS.

Vertebral Artery Surgery

In the 1970s, a Los Angeles vascular surgeon reported that his MS patients showed restoration of lost neurological functions after vertebral artery surgery. He explained that MS was due to clogging of the arteries in the vertebrae of the neck and that his findings before and after surgery would prove this. I was personally appointed by the National Multiple Sclerosis

Society to interview the doctor and review his data. The arteriogram pictures he had were unreadable and the case studies disappointing. Although many patients claimed they had improvements, their postoperative exams showed no change in their conditions. In May 1987, the surgeon's license to practice medicine was revoked.

Calcium EAP and Related Compounds

Calcium aminoethyl phosphate (calcium EAP), calcium orotate, and phosetamin are part of a therapy advocated for many years by Dr. Hans Nieper of Hanover, Germany, who claims that these compounds act as neurotransmitters that stimulate the central nervous system and also protect the nerves against immune attack while repairing damaged nerve function.

In 1984 the German Multiple Sclerosis Society urgently advised MS patients against this treatment because of the lack of evidence of effectiveness and the false claim that it was the only treatment of MS accepted by the German office of health. It is not accepted in Germany or anywhere else.

The treatment with calcium EAP is by injection, five times a week and then every other day. Phosetamin, calcium orotate, and calcium EAP are also taken daily in pill form. The treatment—combined with regular doses of cortisone (5 to 8 milligrams daily), vitamins, and trace elements—must be continued throughout the patient's lifetime. Certain drugs and a raw food diet supplement the therapy.

Experts view the treatments at the Nieper clinic with overwhelming skepticism. The only clinical work on this therapy was reported in 1966 in Aachen, Germany. This study showed that movement disturbances improved in about 32 percent of cases, but no other symptoms were helped. Soon after, calcium EAP treatment was discontinued at the clinic that reported the study.

Until Nieper provides more substantial evidence of its effectiveness, this expensive treatment is not recommended.

In conclusion, rest and steroid treatment, along with the elimination of underlying infections, are the only treatments that have stood the test of time and can get most patients out of an acute attack. While many experimental therapies show great promise for treating and altering the course of MS, how effective they are won't be known until we have the results of research programs now in progress. For now, the greatest successes in treatment have been the tackling of individual symptoms. With rare exception, every symptom of MS can be treated, and every single patient can be improved.

8

Sharpening Your Emotional Tools

> We who are disabled need not apologize for our existence, our rights, our needs, our contributions, our love, our independence, our citizenship, our humanity.
>
> —William Roth, political scientist

The neurologist is the mainstay in handling all your medical symptoms, but only you can tackle the day-to-day obstacles the world places in your way. With MS an entirely new level of challenges appears amid the challenges already accepted as facts of life. Aside from balancing career, family, social, financial, and the ordinary problems of everyday life, you must now cope with the difficulties of MS.

Some people ultimately accept life's challenges more gracefully than others. But, from the first symptoms through the diagnosis and the series of attacks and remissions, few people have any preparation for MS. For most people with MS, the greatest challenges are not the medical ones but the emotional ones. Fear, not MS, can be the greatest crippler of young adults.

In reality, no one can fully prepare you for the emotional

duel with MS. Learning about some of the more common psychological factors involved may help you win the battle. Sharpening your own emotional skills will help you win the war.

The emotional stages after diagnosis of a chronic disease such as MS are very similar to those gone through by the terminally ill, as described by Dr. Elisabeth Kübler-Ross in her book *On Death and Dying*. First there is shock, followed by denial, bargaining, anger, depression, and, ultimately, acceptance. For the terminally ill, death follows acceptance. For the chronically ill, acceptance must last a lifetime. With MS this can be thirty or forty years or more. Acceptance can come more easily when there is a remission—a long period of stability, a return to normal, and full readjustment Then, when MS appears again with a new attack or worsening of an old symptom, the emotional cycle can start all over again.

Although it can be an emotional roller coaster, you can put yourself in charge of the ride. This doesn't mean following terrible clichés like, "Plan for the worst and hope for the best." When a doctor told that to Shirley MacLaine in *Terms of Endearment*, she replied, "And people let you get away with that?" We feel the same way about such haggard advice. Preparing yourself emotionally means learning about your feelings and dealing with them. It means turning up the volume and listening to your innermost thoughts. It means saving up your emotional strength and drawing on it when you most need it. But it also means taking MS out of your life when you're feeling fine.

As with the physical aspects of MS, different stages of the disease have their own unique emotional problems. The newly diagnosed patient will need a different coping strategy from the person who has had MS for ten years or more. The person experiencing the second attack may hit a more serious emotional crisis than with the first or the third. And, just as no two patients seem to have the same physical signs and symptoms, no two patients will react the same either. We can only describe some of the most universal feelings and suggest some ways to cope with them.

Shock

The first shock is the diagnosis. Exactly how a patient handles this depends not only on his or her personality but also on the doctor's. Unfortunately, difficulties are often compounded by misconceptions carried by family and friends, who are capable of making the shock worse. Because of this, it is best to involve as few people as possible.

Ideally, the doctor giving the diagnosis should have evaluated the patient's personality and made the discussion appropriate for the individual. One patient may find more comfort in hearing clinical details of the disease. Another may cope better without hearing any. The advertising executive may need to address her fear of losing the edge in her competitive world. A newlywed may need to talk about the possibility of future pregnancy. Unfortunately, the diagnosis is rarely handled this way. Usually the doctor has a stereotyped speech that is used for every patient.

When a doctor does not tailor the discussion directly to the patient's need, the impact of the diagnosis will be influenced more by the doctor's own personality than by the facts. One of my own patients, on seeking a second opinion on her diagnosis, met with a neurologist who held her MRI pictures up to a window, shook his head from side to side, and said, "This is certainly a bummer," adding, "You should plan on a shortened career and trouble walking by age fifty." In fact, this patient who was thirty-two years old at the time, had thirteen out of thirteen indicators for a good prognosis (discussed in chapter 4). This neurologist could never be mistaken for an optimist, and he didn't even suggest the possibility of scientific breakthroughs that might occur in the eighteen years before she turns fifty.

There are doctors who are too gloomy, too cheerful, too pessimistic, and too optimistic. Too much of anything is not healthy. So, if at all possible, try to evaluate the doctor's personality type. But also be aware that it's very common for a patient initially to resent a doctor who is the bearer of "bad news." "He's an idiot, an uncaring, insensitive person who really doesn't know what he's talking about." This is a normal reaction that shouldn't count in the real evaluation of the doctor. The only true black mark that is deserved at this stage is if the doctor writes MS off as an untreatable disease, which it is not.

As with any other relationship, the patient and doctor must have a courtship, during which they get to know each other, and then a marriage, during which they must trust each other. At the core is good communication, letting each know what they expect from the other. This relationship is going to last a lifetime, so it's important that patient and doctor are compatible and that the doctor's personality will help ease the patient's anxiety, not intensify it.

Emotional Impact of New Technology

Today's MRI-diagnosed patient experiences a greater shock because of the quickness of the diagnosis. This type of shock is not the kind that is going to induce a heart attack. It is a more passive shock; the person is not able to get a grip on exactly what it all means and what to do about it, entering an "I-can't-believe-this-is-happening" state. Many newly diagnosed patients are not ready to identify the problem, talk about it, wrestle with it, or deal with it. They are numbed by it. Since this phenomenon is so new, few doctors today are prepared to handle the "quickly" diagnosed patient. Before the MRI, it took much longer to make an MS diagnosis, and people had more time to get used to the idea. Many patients would actually make the diagnosis before the doctor. They'd go to the library, do their own research, and tell the neurologist of their suspicions. Ultimately, many were relieved to find out they weren't crazy.

The MRI diagnosis has created more profound shock. Pearl Rapp, a social worker who facilitated therapy groups for newly diagnosed patients at the Neuropsychiatric Institute at UCLA, described one clear indication of the change:

> *With each new group, I organize one meeting where medical experts are on hand to answer questions. I encourage group members to invite as many guests as they want—husbands, wives, brothers, sisters, parents, children, anybody. In the past, each member would bring a minimum of two or three guests to the research lecture. The new groups are different. This year, only one person brought one guest. I believe it is the shock of the MRI diagnosis.*

Although the MRI is new to doctors and patients of this MS generation, it is not a bad trade-off. This shock is still better than suffering through the strain of not knowing what is causing the symptoms or thinking that one is crazy. The shock may now last longer, but it won't last forever. It just has to take its own natural course. One way of lessening the shock is to learn as much as possible about MS as quickly as possible. Reading good literature will help diminish the fear and preconceived ideas about MS. Unfortunately, much of the material available is either dated or gloomier than necessary—books and articles picturing people with MS in wheelchairs and such. Be aware that much of the available information is lopsided and often overly dramatic or "inspirational."

The patient must also be cautious of selective listening or reading. This is where your own personality type may come into play. The "Pollyanna" may choose to retain only the most optimistic of statements and will be convinced that he or she is among the percentage of benign cases never to have a second attack. You can hope or pray that's your case, but convincing yourself you'll be that lucky will only set you up for a more dangerous emotional upheaval with the onset of a new sign or symptom. On the other hand, the "Skeptic" only remembers the worst cases written up in academic textbooks. This is just as bad. The person who is sure something horrible is going to happen will diminish his or her quality of life long before any aspect of MS will.

The only way to work toward acceptance and face the emotional challenge of MS is to learn what may or may not happen and then believe that you will be able to face future challenges if and when they happen.

Denial

You may also go through a period of denial, refusing to believe the diagnosis. The doctor must be wrong. He read the tests incorrectly. It can't possibly be true. You might not even feel that sick. Denial is very normal. It's part of your inner self telling you "things shouldn't turn out this bad." Some people don't go through it at all or just have minor hints of denial, like the patient who, while discussing the diagnosis with her boyfriend, suddenly couldn't remember what MS stood for. Although she knew, for that brief moment her subconscious was busy blocking out "multiple sclerosis."

Another common form of denial is seen when a patient

starts looking for a doctor who will come up with a different diagnosis. By all means get a second opinion, and ask the doctor as many questions as you can possibly think of, such as what other possible diseases could cause your symptoms and how they were ruled out. But if your diagnosis conforms to the standard criteria and a board certified neurologist has given you a "definite" MS diagnosis, especially with an MRI confirmation, you're going to have to believe you have MS—no matter how hard it is to swallow.

While denial is a normal part of the adjustment process, sometimes it can have more serious consequences. For instance, it can present itself in the form of forgetting or refusing to take a prescribed treatment. Some people go a step further and develop a devil-may-care attitude, as when a person with a bout of optic neuritis refuses to believe he or she shouldn't drive. Denial, by its very nature, is the phase that's most difficult to recognize. The denial phase can go hand in hand with a refusal to talk about it or even think about it. You may fill your social calendar as if nothing has happened or find yourself changing the subject when others want to discuss it. If others are intervening, try your best to listen with an open mind. Most likely they'll help you learn to deal with the diagnosis.

Denial is not in your best interests and should be distinguished from what we call "healthy denial," which is a person's conscious choice not to think about MS or dwell on the disease every day. Healthy denial can only be accomplished after acceptance has taken place.

BARGAINING

Bargaining, along with guilt, is another common reaction to a diagnosis. Scientists may not know what causes MS, but they do know you didn't get it because you were a bad person or because you cheated on a math test or on your mate. You didn't get MS because you deserve it, and it's not going to go away because you're ready to repent and dedicate your life to helping underprivileged children. This is often a point at which some people test their religious convictions. With moral support, regardless of the source, most people will come to terms with this phase fairly quickly.

Anger

Anger doesn't always follow in the sequence we've outlined. You don't necessarily have to seek out a second (or third or fourth) opinion, deny the diagnosis, bargain with the devil, and then throw a temper tantrum. Whenever it sinks in that you can't pull another piece of paper out of the hat, that you've got multiple sclerosis, you're gonna be mad as hell about it. Good, you should be. You've got big plans and this, you can be sure, certainly doesn't fit in. You're either in love or would like to be. You either have a good job or were trying to get a better one. And now this!

Even if you've had Marcus Welby, M.D., hold your hand through the diagnosis, and even if you have Brad Pitt (or Natalie Portman) vow to stick with you forever, you're going to be angry. You've just been told you have a disease that might or might not be so bad, that can come and go at its own discretion, and for which there is now no cure. (If that doesn't make you mad, check your pulse to see if you're alive!) The bottom line is, you're really mad that MS had to come along and screw up your plans. In fact, dreams you never even had before just got ruined.

If it makes you want to scream, you should. Don't try it in

a crowded elevator or when everyone in the house is asleep. But if it's 2:00 a.m. and you are tempted to tiptoe out of the house, get in the car, and roll all the windows up—let loose. You've got to "ventilate" that anger.

If screaming isn't your thing but crying is, have the best cry you've ever had. Maybe your mate needs this too. Whether it's alone or together, you must grieve. This might feel really painful or even stupid, especially if you're used to keeping a stiff upper lip, but it's not as tough as when you bury your feelings. Let it all hang out. When no one's around, smash a few dishes if it feels good, punch the mattress a few times, or throw a few shoes at the wall. Get that anxiety out of your system. It's healthy.

Anger can manifest itself in many ways. Not everyone shows anger through yelling or kicking a tire. Some people are "passively" angry—they become quiet or withdrawn. They seethe silently or grind their teeth in their sleep. Anger over MS can manifest itself in other areas of your life. You suddenly can't stand the color you painted the garage door last spring; the doctor had no right to keep you waiting for your appointment so long; the waiter was so slow, he didn't deserve even half the tip you left him. These things might all be valid, but you're not really angry about them—you're angry at your MS.

Although these signs of anger are less obvious than others, they still reveal a need to blow off some steam. If you don't take charge of it, you'll find it will come out anyway, usually directed at someone who doesn't deserve the outburst. Misdirected anger isn't fair to the person who bears the brunt of it, whether it's your lover, your mother-in-law, or the poor gas station attendant who didn't wash your window fast enough. And although your MS diagnosis may have given you a right to be angry, the rest of the world isn't going to be tolerant forever. Identify your anger, get rid of it as soon as possible, and move on with the coping process.

Depression

Depression is certainly a reasonable response to an MS diagnosis. If this isn't a reason to be depressed, then what is? Suddenly *unpredictable* becomes the dirtiest word in the English language. You may feel very low, sad, or burdened, as if the weight of the world is on your shoulders. But depression doesn't always have a long face. Sometimes depression shows up disguised as fatigue. You get exhausted, take to bed, sleep a lot. This fatigue can be distinguished from the symptomatic fatigue of MS, which is shorter in duration and usually hits at the same time each day or after overexertion.

You may even think about suicide. You might wonder how many people would come to your funeral and how sorry they'll feel for you. Although morbid, this is not uncommon. These thoughts are normal and usually temporary. In all medical literature there are almost no cases of people who committed suicide because of MS. As people learn more about MS, they learn it is simply not a disease that's worth killing oneself over.

Recently I diagnosed a young female law student. By her second visit she had told me if there was no cure within five years, she was going to kill herself. In the meantime, however, she continued law school. Within a couple of months she was no longer focusing on her five-year suicide plan. And I firmly believe that whether there is a cure in five years or not, she's going to be a fine lawyer. I do not mean to minimize her depression—it was very real and very painful. And in the event that she has a subsequent attack, she may harbor such thoughts again. But working toward that degree will keep her in control of her life.

(At this point it's important to say that general thoughts about suicide are normal. Plotting out any details or taking any action is not. If you've taken any step, such as storing pills or organizing a plan, please seek professional help immediately. Your MS is probably the straw breaking the camel's back, and you need to sort out the other problems in your life that preceded your diagnosis.)

Now that you know that depression is normal, what should you do about it? First of all, don't pop a pill and mask it. Don't hide it or deny it. Try to understand it and live with it for a while. Go through this phase, no matter how painful. Don't let friends drag you out to cheer you up right away. You need to go through a grieving period. Others may mean well, but sometimes the best way to get over depression is to have a friend just sit by your side, get you a tissue when you shed a tear, and just stare out the window with you. Just know that depression is part of the healing process and that you are going to feel emotionally stronger very soon. Right now you feel as if you're never going to be happy again. But be patient—you will be. It may be hard to believe now, but you are resilient, and you are going to bounce back when you're ready.

The person actively adjusting to MS will eventually get fed up with feeling depressed and move on to acceptance. If you feel frustrated that you are not progressing toward this goal, consult your neurologist, who may suggest counseling, medication, or both.

ACCEPTANCE

How will you know if you have arrived at an emotionally healthy acceptance? Here is our ten-point checklist:

1. MS is no longer the focus of your life.
2. Depression, anger, and bitterness are occasional emotions, not a way of life.
3. Although you are optimistic, you accept that you may have either a mild or more progressive course in the future.
4. You continue to make plans for the future, with the understanding that they may need to be altered.
5. In the event of physical impairment, you are able to readjust goals in work, leisure-time activities, and relationships to match ability.
6. You are no longer fearful of the future.
7. You are willing to accept help from others graciously while finding your own way to reciprocate.
8. Regardless of physical limitations, you maintain a positive self-image.
9. You follow good health practices and avoid tempting fate with aggravating factors.
10. You view MS as an added burden in your life, not the reason for all your problems.

The emotional phases we've adapted from Dr. Elisabeth Kübler-Ross, along with our ten-point checklist of acceptance, are just guidelines to use for understanding the emotional upheaval you've been through or the one you're still going through. Most likely, at least one key person in your life has been involved from the diagnosis stage. By now you've learned if this person can be helpful or not. In the best of circumstances, this person will hold your hand when you need it, give reassurance when it's called for, listen when you need to talk, and inspire independence when that's appropriate. Unfortunately, not everyone has such a friend or relative. More often than not, we are stuck with overbearing mothers, fragile spouses, friends who mean well but say the wrong things, and even friends who disappear when things get sticky.

Well, MS *does* get sticky, and only you know if you need more help in coping. Often, a person with MS chooses to diminish the role of the disease in everyday life and seeks counseling with a social worker, psychologist, or psychiatrist, or joins a support group. This can be valuable, as it keeps the focus on MS at a set time and place; ideally, you will learn to "leave MS in the therapist's office."

THE SECOND ATTACK

You've already gone through the Kübler-Ross stages of shock, denial, bargaining, anger, depression, and acceptance. It may be a year, two years, even five years since your onset, and things have been going really well. Occasionally you had a pang of fear that a new attack would come along and muck up your plans. But you took that vacation, you had that great romance, and nothing was spoiled. You were almost convinced that the rest of your course would be silent, but dammit, it's here again.

Emotionally, the second attack can be more difficult than the first. With your first exacerbation, you were probably too scared or worried to understand the implications of the actual attack. After your diagnosis you learned about MS and went through all the stages of acceptance. But was it really full acceptance? If your symptoms disappeared and your life got back to normal, acceptance may have been more in theory—especially with a remitting-relapsing course and a clean bill of health from the neurologist. But now you have new symptoms, and you are wondering all over again. "Why is this happening to me?" Now that you're more knowledgeable, you're also asking, "How severe will this attack be?

How long will it last? Will I fully recover? Will this mark the change in my course?"

The second attack is often the time when the realization of MS really sinks in. Just hang in there. You will probably go through another Kübler-Ross cycle. You may be less shocked, more angry, equally depressed. Give it some time. Get bed rest right away, and follow the other treatments your neurologist prescribes. See how you respond. You'll bounce back completely to normal. The second attack will probably be a worse emotional blow than the first. But think of its being a little like the first time someone broke your heart. Take comfort that you'll toughen up and it will never hurt quite as much again. It may hurt again, but at least MS will become the devil you know.

Don't lose hope. Although you may continue to have MS attacks throughout your life, you may still find yourself in long periods of remission. McAlpine reported an extraordinary case of a man who was diagnosed as having MS at age twenty-four during a nine-month episode of weakness in the leg and bladder trouble. A few years later he had numbness in the hands. He had no other problems and remained symptom-free until age seventy-one when he developed paresthesias in his right hand and foot. We don't advise convincing yourself that you won't have another attack for forty years or so—many people have frequent attacks early in the course of their MS. But you will learn to cope. Get tough and be optimistic. Remember that each symptom can be treated, and there's a very good chance you will return to normal.

Emotional Impact of a Progressive Course

So far, we've walked you through the emotional stages of MS from the moment of diagnosis to subsequent attacks. We've talked about the emotional impact of MS when the person returns to normal or nearly to normal. For the 10 to 20 percent of people who begin MS with a chronic-progressive course, acceptance is much more difficult. The emotional phases still follow the Kübler-Ross pattern, but acceptance must be made without the benefit of a remission of symptoms or a return to normal. This, more than any other form, will test a person's mettle. This is also a challenge for those with a remitting-relapsing course that has turned progressive. Uncertainty prevails as to when the MS will stabilize.

Although a number of people with primary-progressive MS will remain ambulatory, able to get around with or without walking aids, for many others permanent loss of mobility is the reality to which they must adjust, and this is a tough hand to be dealt. But it is still not the end of the world. If you're motivated, you can figure out how to continue to lead a productive life. When people are really honest about their feelings, they admit that they are really not afraid of life in a wheelchair but of alienation, loneliness, job discrimination, and other such barriers to a normal life. The truth is that success in tackling MS is not determined by mobility so much as it is by attitude and personality. Ask yourself if you'd rather spend time with someone who is witty and charming and in a wheelchair or someone who is dull, bitter, and can jog around the block. As you sharpen your emotional skills, you'll fare better if you also sharpen your interpersonal skills.

If your MS progresses and you lose certain central nervous system functions, you are going to mourn those losses. But you cannot mourn forever. You must find your own way to readjust your life and reemerge. This is probably the greatest test of will and emotional strength you will ever face. While coping with the physical aspects of MS, you must have the presence of mind to make necessary adjustments in such areas as career, financial planning, and relationships—certainly a handful for anyone. Don't try to sort out everything at once. Tackle one problem at a time. Seek the advice of experts. Talk to a financial planning expert, a career counselor, a marriage counselor, and anyone else who can help. Don't wait for a problem to arise—you must also think in terms of "preventive" emotional medicine.

Remember that there is never just one solution to a problem, and some problems have no great solutions at all. You should only try to find the best solution for your situation. For some, deep religious convictions will help the emotional healing process. For others, involvement in a research program will give renewed hope and optimism. Even without participating in a research program, the person with a progressive course can still feel optimistic. As we'll discuss in detail in chapter 11, when a cure is ultimately discovered, there's a good chance it will benefit everyone. In August 2005, the National MS Society awarded four grants, totaling over $15 million, to study tissue repair and protection in MS. This work is moving toward reversing the damage caused by MS and restoring function to those who have had the disease for years. Recent scientific advances in many different fields, according to the NMSS, have come together to bring the dream of repairing brain tissue within our grasp. Awarded the largest single grants ever by the NMSS, four teams will be led by researchers from Johns Hopkins, University of Wisconsin, Cambridge University, and University College London and they will work with collaborators in Canada, Europe, and the United States.

Who Can Handle MS Best?

There is no personality profile of a person who will cope best with MS. For many, adversity—such as an MS diagnosis and subsequent battles with the disease—helps promote personal growth. So even the person who seems least likely to be able to cope with MS may turn out to be the one who marks the greatest personal triumphs.

MS is a kick in the gut that will no doubt change your life. You may feel a loss of innocence, a lot less carefree, but there's a positive side to the drama too. MS forces you to look at what your true goals are. If there's something you really want to do, you'll do it now. You've learned that nothing should wait till tomorrow. You'll make every day count. Crazy things will make you happy. What the rest of the world takes for granted, you will start to celebrate. MS interferes with brain signals, but there are still plenty of things going on that you can control. The only loss to prove a real tragedy would be the loss of your sense of humor. It has been said that in MS, your sense of humor may not be the first to go, but it's the toughest to live without.

9

MS and Your Relationships

Multiple sclerosis obviously affects your relationships with other people, from your lover or spouse to your parents, children, friends, co-workers, employers, and doctor. Whom to tell and when and how to tell them are just a few of the issues MS raises. So few people understand what multiple sclerosis is, let alone understand its emotional impact, that it's up to you to facilitate healthy relationships. You know what you're thinking and feeling. You can't expect others to read your mind or to act appropriately at all times. Those closest to you may be going through their own anxious reactions to your MS. And those beginning new relationships with you may feel varying levels of discomfort. Don't write scripts of how you'd like others to be. Accept MS as your burden and accept that you'll try your best to make your relationships work.

Disclosure

As a general rule, we believe MS is best kept a private matter, not a public tragedy. The fewer people you tell, the easier it will be to diminish the importance of MS in your life. If you remove the temptation to talk about it all the time, you will force your focus to change. You're not under any obligation to share all your problems with all of your friends. You censor other areas of your personal life and keep various people on a need-to-know basis; the same rules apply to your MS.

Still, from time to time, you will need someone to talk to. Some people prefer talking to more than one friend, so they don't feel they're a burden to any one person. But whether it's one friend or more is up to you. Just be sure you make the right choice. From that moment on, you're in control of who knows what and when. Take stock of your relationships. You probably won't want to involve a friend who has a habit of topping every story with a bigger tale. And you probably wouldn't choose someone who talks in platitudes like, "Something good will come out of this; it always does." The basic rule is to rely only on people you could rely on in the past. Be honest with yourself. Many of us spend our lives trying to make relationships into something they never were in the first place. Your "ex" is not finally going to show some compassion just because you really need a shoulder to lean on. Your self-centered sister is not suddenly going to undergo a personality change and realize you're the one who needs some love and attention right now. She may for a moment, but people are who they are. Self-centered people ultimately react as if everything is happening to them. (Your sister may be so overcome with depression on your behalf that she has to take to bed for a week. This may appear to be out of deep feeling for you, but it really makes her the object of others' worry.)

The emotional crisis periods of MS will make you take a good look at those around you. Your choice of whom to turn to should not become an exercise to weed out who belongs in your life and who doesn't. Your life should be full of different kinds of people on different levels of intimacy. One person might be the friend who shares your interest in old Hitchcock thrillers. Another might be your aunt who bakes a great blueberry pie but doesn't quite "get it." Such people are not meant to share your deepest, darkest secrets—they are meant to share experiences. If, on the other hand, this overall evaluation has made you realize that a particular relationship needs repair, do so, but only after your crisis has passed.

The question of disclosure of your MS may come up at many different times, because of a variety of situations—a new job, the bonding of a new friendship, or a serious love affair. We'll take these situations and more on an individual basis, but there is one general guideline. The key question to ask yourself in deciding whom to tell is, Why am I telling him or her? You should know in your heart if you're making the right decision. Here are some examples, each starting with the implicit words *I'm revealing my MS because.*

- We've fallen in love and it's only fair to bring it out in the open.
- Not telling has created a sense of alienation and a barrier to our relationship.
- If my boss could understand why I need a more flexible work schedule, I could do my job better.
- If that person knew what my life was really like, he (or she) wouldn't have done that.
- If that person knew what challenges I face, he (or she) would respect me more.
- If the boss only knew what I battle every day, he (or she) would give me a break.

The first three examples—exploring a lifetime commitment, bonding a friendship, or maintaining or advancing your career—are valid reasons for disclosure of your MS. The last three are flimsy reasons at best. If you expect anyone to treat you better, respect you more, or give you a break because you have MS, you are using the disease to manipulate those around you. Instead of telling these people about your MS, work on other interpersonal skills with them, such as communication of fairness, assertiveness, and confrontation. Don't use the disclosure of MS to make another party feel guilty or embarrassed for not treating you better, for revenge, or for undeserved or unwarranted special treatment. This approach will only backfire in the long run.

DATING AND MS

Dating is tough for everyone, regardless of age, sex, appearance, or status in life. Bookshelves lined with such titles as *Smart Women, Foolish Choices*; *How to Make a Man Fall in Love with You*; and *How to Pick Up Girls* prove it. They sell millions and millions of copies each year to those who want to find the perfect mate. Loneliness is a national crisis in the United States, and for the single person with MS, finding a loving mate may seem an impossible feat. It is not. I very recently counseled two patients who brought their new fiancés to my office. They have the same chances of a successful marriage as anyone else—maybe better. These couples made a serious commitment to each other. What was their secret? There's no ten-point plan to falling in love despite adversity. But there is a key to getting the relationship off to a good start.

If your MS has visible symptoms (your walk may be unsteady, perhaps, and this will be apparent to others) you will have to discuss it with anyone you date right away. If you don't initiate the discussion, your date may suspect such problems as drinking or substance abuse. So it's best to get things out in the open right away. As in the development of other social skills, such as asking someone out on a date or developing a sexual rapport, you will ultimately develop your own philosophy and understanding of what feels most comfortable for you. One of the simplest ways of handling the situation is to tell your date that you have a mild neurological problem. If he or she asks no more questions, don't volunteer anything. If there is a specific follow-up, such as "What is it?" answer directly that you have nothing contagious, just a mild case of MS that comes and goes. You might want to reinforce that you feel great and, by the way, are having a wonderful time on the date. Keep the conversation as short and general as possible and avoid going into clinical details. The more "medical" you sound, the more serious your date may think the problem is—you will risk sounding the alarm button before he or she has a chance to learn how witty and charming you are. You can easily change the subject by explaining that although you personally find MS interesting, you don't want to be like your Aunt Sophie who could talk about her appendix operation for hours on end. As the relationship develops, you'll have time to share your innermost feelings, but the first date is neither the time nor the place.

For people with mild or invisible MS, disclosure to a dating partner can and probably should wait. MS is not contagious, so there is certainly no moral or ethical reason for disclosure. And it's more important for people to get to know who you are, not what you have. Other people don't tell you their health history on the first date, so don't feel obligated to present yourself as, "Hi-my-name-is-Joanna-and-I-have-MS." The truth is that most people, even the most educated, know very little about MS. If you don't have to bring it into a budding relationship, don't. The emphasis at these times is best put on romance and shared experiences. You'll know from other indicators if your partner is one who will provide a good shoulder to lean on. See how he or she responds in other day-to-day problems. How compassionate is he or she? How does he or she respond when you talk about a rotten day at the office?

Test the waters by telling your partner about another personal problem that comes up in your life. One of my patients decided to tell her boyfriend about an ongoing feud over her grandfather's will. When she began to discuss the situation, her boyfriend replied, "I'm sorry, but I really don't think you should discuss this outside of your family." He just didn't want to hear about it. She knew he was not the type of man with whom she could comfortably discuss her MS, but she continued to see him for a while. Although he had little personal sensitivity, he was an interesting date who made her laugh a lot. Although she knew he was not the one for her in the long run, seeing him was better than sitting home feeling sorry for herself. But she was in control because she had learned to distinguish a "Mr. Right" from a "Mr. Right Now."

Until you find the right mate, you're bound to be involved in a series of relationships that eventually don't work out. This has nothing to do with MS; it has everything to do with the mating process, which can be frightening for anyone. Think about it: You go out to see if you like the other person (and if the other person likes you) well enough to continue. If you tell everyone you date that you have MS, it can become too easy to blame any failures on the disease. When you remove MS from this process, you'll be forced to look at who you are. Are you an interesting date? Are you a good listener? Can you keep up with the conversation? Does your date find you sexually attractive? If you've lost your perspective on such factors, take a good look at your relationships before your diagnosis. Were they better? Don't give yourself a built-in excuse for why they're not working now. Are you still angry about your MS diagnosis? Your anger, not your MS, is going to make you less appealing to a partner.

Some people argue that it's better to get the disclosure out of the way early—they'd rather not invest time, energy, and emotions in a relationship with someone they later learn cannot cope with MS. Disclosure becomes a self-protective measure, like that of the man who won't wear his toupée on the first date. (If a woman is turned off by bald men, there's no reason to make it a surprise later on.) If you have a need for such self-protection, you should not hold off disclosure. But you should also be aware of the consequences of disclosure. Today's courtships are very delicate. People usually discover all the wonderful things about each other first and then learn to deal with each other's flaws. Often relationships begin with incredible fireworks that then fizzle out as quickly as they appeared. On the first or second date, a couple might find themselves in bed exchanging life stories. But then, after three weeks, the magic has disappeared. For the single person who was hoping this might be the relationship that works out, it's deflating. For the single person who has already disclosed MS, it can be devastating. There's no way to know it just wasn't destined to work out anyway. String a few relationship failures in a row, and you'll be convinced that no one will ever love you because you have MS. If you don't tell your partner about your MS, you'll allow the relationship to unfold more naturally and succeed or fail on its own merits.

Your mating problems probably have absolutely nothing to do with your MS. Your MS diagnosis may just have made you take a better look at things. For many, it's a good time to seek counseling to find out if there's been a bad pattern repeated throughout their relationships. You may not be able to fix your MS, but you can still work on your personal growth.

So, date, explore relationships without disclosing your

MS, and don't be afraid to fall in love. Of course, there's a chance you'll have your heart broken, but that rule applied before MS. Don't lead a sheltered life; enjoy the richness of it. If your heart gets broken, you'll deal with that, too. You've already faced a much greater fear.

Many people with MS experience a heightened feeling of vulnerability. They feel more fragile than ever before. Going through the profound experience of an MS diagnosis has probably changed your emotional composition too, but just be yourself. Your increased vulnerability might be more painful to you, but also might make you more attractive to others.

Having everything in your life start to go right can make you feel just as frightened and vulnerable as having everything go wrong. It's not uncommon to feel panicky just when you're on top of the world. When you fall in love and reach the mezzanine between clouds eight and nine, you'll take a deep breath and think, "My MS better not mess up this love affair." It's normal to have these fleeting moments, but bury them. Use every bit of willpower to block them out, and go for the moment. Tell yourself that no matter what happens later, you'll always have this moment of being in love right now. You'll turn around one day and have enough romantic moments strung together to realize you've taken MS out of your romantic life.

When is the right moment for disclosure? When it's time to talk about marriage. Don't wait for a vulnerable moment when you're sure you're going to be abandoned. Don't run away or start acting strange so that your partner is forced to drag it out of you. Plan ahead for the moment, and when you're faced with it, you'll have worked out the kinks and have a better grip on pulling it off confidently. Just as the patient's reaction to MS will often mirror the doctor's attitude at the time of diagnosis, a partner's attitude will mirror that of the person with MS. When you are ready to talk about marriage, emphasize how much you love the other person and that you would like to be married, and then add that you may face certain difficulties in the future. By discussing them, you will learn if you can face them together.

Your partner may or may not have suspected something already, depending on your symptoms, your remission, and other factors. You may have had an attack that you explained with a half-truth. It's important to explain why you didn't reveal your MS sooner. Emphasize that you made a choice not to make MS part of your relationship in the past and that you hope it won't be a part of your relationship in the future.

You must expect that no matter how well prepared you are and how well you handle the situation, your disclosure will be a shock to your partner. After all, he or she is very much in love with you. Don't go into a lot of clinical details right away. Do volunteer love, reinforcement, and confidence in your relationship. Give your partner the option of buying a little time to get used to the idea, as you have. Avoid manipulating by guilt. It's okay to say, "I'm really afraid that this will ruin everything we've built," but open the door to discussion by adding, "but it's better to deal with it now than later." Your partner may withdraw, get angry, or feel betrayed, hostile, or devastated. You've got to be ready for anything. Be tough and reinforce that no matter what, you're both going to get past this moment. Talk about the philosophic points in choosing a mate. Is there any guarantee against cancer, a heart attack, a stroke? Does anyone else really have any guarantees? Most important, address the hope for advancements in treatment and research toward a cure. Then lend your partner this book.

Finally, be prepared to let go. Although you have both fallen in love, your partner may simply not be cut out to live with MS and the unpredictable factors in your life. There may be childhood memories of a sickly relative or reasons buried in the subconscious that you'll never know. On the other hand, don't be so prepared for the worst that you push your partner away. Try to hold the relationship together. Suggest premarriage counseling. But, ultimately, accept that this was the risk of disclosure. If you have to let go, let go with dignity. In time, your partner may come back with a new spirit or a new perspective. If not, you'll have to start over. None of this is easy, but if it's your goal to live happily ever after, you're going to have to try again. You'll eventually find someone with one other reaction—understanding.

MS AND YOUR SPOUSE

MS is going to have an impact on your marriage. When you exchanged vows to love and honor each other in sickness and in health, you probably thought that test would come in your sunset years. But it's here now and you have to cope with it.

Management of MS in a marriage requires patience and understanding—qualities important to any marriage. And, presumably, you have a foundation of love and respect. You must also now sharpen your skills of communication and negotiation because your roles may have to change from time to time.

If your MS is in remission, there may be no problem to face but that of fatigue. As we've discussed, fatigue is a difficult symptom for another person to understand. You may look healthy, but you peter out before the end of the day. Although treatments help a lot of people a lot of the time, they don't help everybody all of the time. If you've done your best to organize your day for maximum efficiency and you're still fatigued, you must help your spouse to understand that you can no longer do your share of duties. To make sure you don't neglect your spouse, it's important to let the car get dirty or the laundry pile up from time to time. You may think about redefining your chores. It may work out better if the person with MS trades paying the bills for vacuuming or trades organizing the tax receipts for cleaning out the garage.

When you're in a new attack, for one or two weeks or maybe as long as six, you may need your mate to help take over shopping, cooking, mowing the lawn, washing the car, cleaning up, and caring for the children. In temporary situations like this, it is ideal for the welfare of you and your marriage to hire extra help. The maintenance of a small emergency fund for times like this will really help. It may reap benefits you can't put a price on. Sometimes the spouse is a wonderful person but just not in the particular role he or she is being asked to fill. Don't force it; hire someone to take over the chore.

The most patience and understanding is needed when a person with MS becomes disabled. This is a real test of love. If the marriage has not been a strong one or a variety of problems is eating away at it, the disability can become an excuse for ending it. Look at the marriage problems you had before the MS diagnosis and deal with them. Don't expect your partner to feel guilty enough about your MS to correct whatever was wrong. That can only work as a short-term remedy.

Although at this point it is undocumented, there does seem to be a high divorce rate in MS marriages. This fact may hide the many other woes that beset a marriage. Some believe that more men than women leave a spouse with MS. This is probably true and may be due to the fact that women are traditionally more comfortable in the role of nurturer. But if true love is there, MS, with or without disability, can be conquered by the husband and wife working together. It is encouraging to see how many good marital relationships there are and how many spouses continue to care for the loved one through all adversities. It is also possible that health care professionals talk more to couples in trouble. Happy couples keep more to themselves.

What do these couples have that creates a lasting relationship? We have found five key elements to a successful MS marriage:

1. These couples face facts early in the game. They find out what is likely to happen, accept it, and make plans to deal with it, thus taking the fear of the unknown out of the marriage.
2. They get help from family, neighbors, friends, and health care workers when needed to weather fatigue, attacks, or disability.
3. The person with MS turns the medical problems over to the doctor, not the spouse. It can be very wearing to hear medical complaints day after day. There is nothing the partner can do but feel guilty, sorrowful, and helpless. Information can, of course, be shared, but those who are selective maintain stronger relationships.
4. They learn to take the MS out of the relationship. They go out at night, visit friends, and take trips and romantic vacations. They find ways to do each and every activity together in spite of MS.
5. Finally, the couples with the greatest success never let the sexual side of the marriage deteriorate. They realize there are many reasons why sexual activity may decline over the years. If things have become stale, they use creativity and imagination to bring romance back into the relationship. They analyze the variety of reasons why one partner may have lost interest—emotional depression, financial burdens, midlife personality change, and more. Or they find out if the partner

> who has lost interest has a legitimate gripe. Has the mate become less appealing in dress, appearance, or use of language or behavior? There are many reasons for the decline of sexual activity in a marriage. Do not assume it's MS. Of course, a small percentage of people develop sexual dysfunction in MS. In all such cases, however, something can be done, as discussed in chapter 7.

Ultimately, if you decide you need a marriage counselor, examine your marriage before MS, look at the problems you have now, and discuss MS, but do not focus on it as the root of all your trouble.

MS and Your Children

Children, with their keen intuitive sense, will have figured out that something is wrong with Mom or Dad long before they are told. Even if MS is invisible, children are incredibly sensitive to changes in the household atmosphere. No matter what age the children are, if they are old enough to talk with, they are old enough to be informed that a parent has MS.

As in many other crises, such as divorce or a death in the family, the young child may not have the maturity to understand what it means fully. Often, the child will think that anything bad that has happened in the house is his or her fault—if he or she had been better behaved this would have never happened. It should be explained and reinforced that the child is in no way responsible; no one is, for that matter. Try not to explain MS in terms of a disease that you just get and no one knows how you get it. This can fuel a child's vivid imagination to believe that he or she could wake up one day with something just like it. Emphasize that young children do not get MS, only much older people. And, unlike measles, mumps, or the flu, no one else in the family is going to catch it.

As the parent with MS goes through various MS stages and adjustments, children must be continually involved in the family communication. With each attack, you must reinforce that you may not be feeling well but you're going to be okay. If you must go to the hospital for treatment, be honest with the children. Talk to them on the phone regularly or send notes home. Be on the lookout for warning signs that a child is experiencing emotional difficulties. Clues include nightmares, changes in eating habits, loss of interest in school or after-school activities, and changes in personality such as withdrawal or negative attitudes. (For the disabled parent of a younger child, there are dolls with a variety of disabilities that help open difficult communication lines. By watching the child play with such dolls, the parent can often learn the child's deepest, darkest thoughts. Then it's up to you to address the problem.)

With teenagers communication about MS should be direct and include the same reassurances that would be given a younger child. But you should be very sensitive to how well you are communicating. Younger children seem to be more honest if they don't understand something. But if a teenager is asked if he or she understands what is being said, he or she might be inclined to answer yes just to avoid embarrassment or make things easier. Older children might also harbor anger toward you and your MS, or they may feel self-conscious about you, which can be very painful. Suddenly, they forget to tell you about a PTA meeting or talent show. Hang in there. Don't forget that this is the same teenager who thinks a little pimple is a valid reason to stay home from school for three days. There's a good chance your teenager was going to act like this toward you even if MS had never entered the picture. Teenagers are self-conscious about the way their parents dress, the corny things their parents say, the unhip ways they think. Realize, too, that there are good kids and not-so-good kids. Many are a bit of both until they mature into adults. The key to raising great kids is for the parent with MS to remain emotionally healthy. If you can get rid of your own anger, fears, and hostility, your children are less likely to adopt negative attitudes.

Don't worry about how your MS will affect the lives of your children later. If you help them remove fear and anger, facing adversity will mature them. They will learn stronger values early. As they are asked to take on more responsibility in the house, they will learn to be more responsible than their peers. You are not abandoning your children. You will be there to discipline them, mold them, and give them love and encouragement.

If you feel that you'd be a better parent if you didn't have MS, you're doing something wrong. You're not being creative or resourceful enough. If you have to miss a football game, have a mini pep rally or victory celebration at home. See if you can get a DVD of the game and watch it, play by play, with the family. Don't think that because you missed the football game, you should say yes when your son asks to stay out until 3:00 a.m. Guilt is no basis for family decisions. It's not a bad idea to ask yourself, What would I say if I didn't have MS?

Finally, don't let anyone tell your children how to interact with you. A well-meaning friend or relative might tell a more difficult child not to give you a hard time or not to be so rebellious. This will usually backfire. During different stages in a child's life, he or she will go through moments or phases. It may zap your energy at times, but a child who's going through a rebellious phase will do it more secretively if told to behave just to make life easier on you. You may have MS, but this doesn't mean your kids won't give you a run for your money. You really don't want them obeying you because they think you're fragile. You want them obeying you because you've taught them right from wrong. Make sure you and your spouse are on the lookout for this.

But don't be a martyr either. Let your children know your levels of adjustment to MS. If you keep communication open, you're more likely to raise children who are sensitive to how you are feeling and when it's appropriate to challenge you. They will learn to face issues appropriately. And they will develop the kind of sixth sense that later lets them ask the boss for that raise at just the right time.

As children get older, it's normal to fear the day they will leave the nest. Most parents go through this. The parent with MS, however, may feel it that much more. Fight this yourself. If you have built a good relationship with your children, they won't let you down when you need them. So don't clutch too hard. You've got to let them get out and experience the world. If you pull the reins too tight, they will learn to resent you. If your home is full of happy memories and laughter, it is a place to which they will always be glad to return.

MS and Your Parents

The age at which MS commonly strikes is a delicate one for most parent-child relationships. Many newly diagnosed people are experiencing their first independence—they may have even started their own families. The complicated process of cutting the invisible umbilical cord with parents had finally ended or was nearing an end, and a sudden uncomfortable feeling of dependency reemerges. The roles you fought so hard to define through young adulthood appear to be in jeopardy. The overbearing parent may try to strengthen his or her turf. Or perhaps the elderly parent who was learning to depend on you is sent into a tailspin panic. Whatever the case, the parent-child relationship is one more part of your life affected by MS. But before you get more frustrated at the disease, remind yourself that every event in your life altered your relationship with your parents. Remember getting your own apartment, dating a person they didn't approve of, marrying someone they didn't think was good enough, getting divorced and hearing, "I told you so," or taking a job out of town. You've been redefining your relationship with your parents your whole adult life. If you choose to tell them about your MS—and this is by no means mandatory—you are about to enter another phase.

In some situations you may be pleasantly surprised to find they bring comfort and nurturing. In others you may find yourself beating back their tendency to get overinvolved in your life, your decisions, and your health management. As with all your relationships, you are going to have to learn to assert yourself. You don't have to grin and bear everything because they are your parents who love you and mean well. In fact, because they *are* your parents, they're going to love you anyway, so if you need to learn how to assert yourself better, you might as well start now. If they treat you as if you're twelve years old again, you've got to say, "I appreciate what you're saying, but you should know it doesn't make me feel very good when you say it." Or if they get overly upset, let them know it doesn't help you to watch them wring their hands in worry.

On the other hand, don't get overly independent just because you don't like accepting their help. If you are fortunate enough to have parents who can make life easier on you from time to time, take advantage of it. Give yourself a break. It might help your overall health status in the long run.

MS and Your Friends

Good friendships do not happen by accident. They're cultivated with loving care. You've cultivated a few prior to MS, and you'll cultivate some along the way. Cultivating means you must be a good friend back. When you enjoy periods of good health, you'll remember to extend yourself to those friends you can call on when you need to. Many times friends of a person with MS feel they can't impose by asking a favor. You may have to encourage them or volunteer to help them. It doesn't have to be a big favor, just a thoughtful one like, "There's a great sale on pantyhose at the mall today. I'm headed over there this afternoon. Can I pick you up a few pairs?" Thinking of others in this way will make you feel less self-conscious asking others to do favors when you really need them.

In the process of taking MS out of your marriage, a good friend can come in very handy. For example, if you need some romantic time alone with your mate, a good friend might take the kids off your hands for an evening. This can be extremely important to your marriage, and you can be honest about it with a good friend. Your friends might decide it's not such a bad idea and drop their kids off at your house from time to time.

Don't be overly fearful of burdening your friends. The best friends you have will be calling you to see what they can do when they sense you need a hand. If they don't sense you need a hand, you must learn to ask for one. Friends are friends, not mind readers. They have their own full lives with their own families, other friends, and other responsibilities. They are not spending their free time wondering what they can do for you today. But if they are true friends, they'll be more than happy to lend you a hand if you need one. However, you have to ask. This is one of the biggest problem areas for people who have MS. There is a tendency to "tough it out" rather than ask anything of anyone. This is not an easy issue, but it's one of the more important ones to resolve within yourself. Asking someone's help doesn't have to mean an erosion of your independence—especially if it gives you the energy at the end of the day to have a better quality of life.

With newer friends, if you choose to tell them about your MS, you will have to break the ice and let them know it's okay to talk about it and ask you questions. You should be well-enough adjusted so that you'll have other things in common to talk about. One goal you should keep in mind for your friendships is enriching your life through shared experiences. That means going to museums, dashing out for ice cream or a pizza, or arguing whether or not Richard Nixon has been treated fairly by historians. If you find MS is becoming more and more of a focal point, that the other aspects of your friendships are diminishing in the balance, a weekly support group might give you the emotional outlet you need. This helps confine your focus of MS to a certain time and place, allowing the rest of your life to return to business as usual.

Your Relationship with Your Doctor

One of the most important relationships, yet one of the least cultivated, is that between the patient and doctor. Until a cure for MS is found, this is a relationship that is going to last a long time—so it had better be a good one. It is very important for you to have a doctor who gives you confidence and hope.

The doctor who tells you "there is nothing we can do" or that disability is inevitable, is, frankly, a loser. Find another doctor. Don't ever be afraid to change neurologists.

Your search for "Dr. Right" is important, and you may try out a few relationships before you settle down. The ideal doctor is someone who practices medicine as both a science and an art. This means a doctor who keeps on top of the research and who listens to your symptoms to find a treatment for each and every one. You need a doctor who is available to talk to you when a newspaper or TV station makes some dramatic statement about MS. You'll need to know if each new discovery or breakthrough is legitimate.

Finding such a person is not that easy. At the university or teaching hospital, you'll find top scientists who are doing original research in MS but who don't have the time to get to know the patient well or deal with the daily problems of MS. The doctor in private practice may have the compassion and the right bedside manner but be out of touch with the latest developments. Which doctor you pick depends on your situation. The best bet for the newly diagnosed, the benign case, or one in long remission is to find a good neurologist in private practice. If the attacks are more frequent or a downhill slide begins, and the regular doctor has run out of ideas for treatment, then it's time to find a doctor at a university medical center.

Being a good patient is the other half of the patient-doctor relationship. While you should have a rapport that lets you call the doctor whenever you need, you should not overuse the phone. Don't make every symptom an emergency—it is not. Give a new symptom two or three days before calling. It can, at least, wait until office hours. Prepare for the visit or phone call in advance by making notes on what is important to discuss and what questions you'd like to ask. Remember, no question is too stupid to ask. But you don't want to keep calling the doctor back with "I'm sorry, but I forgot to mention. . . ." Keep notes of your own symptoms and the times and dates they appear and disappear. If you don't discuss each problem regularly, bring the log to your six-month checkup. Take notes when you talk to the doctor so you don't have to call back and ask again. Finally, try not to be the type of patient who bad-mouths every other doctor. You may feel very frustrated over your previous medical care, but each new doctor doesn't want to hear who's on your blacklist. Your medical records will speak for themselves. If your medical care has been horrendous, report it to the American Medical Association. But if it was a situation in which you were just frustrated by MS or your personality was incompatible with the doctor's, there's no reason to broadcast it all over the community.

MS and Your Career

Often it is hard work for the person with MS just to hang on to a job. This has little to do with the person's ability and more to do with the hidden discrimination of the work world. A national survey, conducted by the National Institute of Neurological and Communicative Disorders and Stroke (NINCDS) and published by the U.S. Department of Health and Human Services, found that MS dramatically affects work status. Four out of ten people with MS left the work force or were dismissed from their jobs because of their illness. One out of ten changed jobs because of MS.

The careers of men seemed to be more affected than those of women. While 82 percent of men were working at the onset of MS, only 39 percent were still working at the time of the survey. At the onset of MS, about 46 percent of women were employed. At the time of the survey, that figure had dropped to 40 percent. It is possible that the difference in impact between men and women may be the type of employment at stake. The more traditional male occupations, involving physical labor or the executive suite, may be less accommodating than traditional female occupations. (This is just our speculation, not a conclusion of the NINCDS.)

Other studies in the United Kingdom and West Germany report that 75 to 80 percent of people with MS are unemployed. But researchers report that half of those had both ability and willingness to work. In many cases lack of transportation was the only reason for unemployment.

MS does not by itself mean eventual unemployment. Unfortunately the discrimination and lack of understanding associated with MS can mean just that. Where there are more sophisticated attitudes toward persons with disabilities, more people with MS remain employed. A 1982 study in Israel showed almost 60 percent of people with MS still employed. In England, where a group of postal employees with disabilities were offered alternative positions, a higher percentage of people remained employed than the average for the rest of the country.

Psychological factors can also account for loss of employment. Depression, lack of motivation, and difficulty in coping are acknowledged factors in unemployment. Finally, there are those who accept early retirement and company pensions on diagnosis without any consideration of their own MS prognosis and type of disability. So, while many people with MS find themselves jobless, it's not necessarily the result of any physical aspect of the disease.

This is tragic. Besides the emotional impact, the economic impact of MS is enormous. In 1976 the U.S. government estimated that the total lifetime financial loss per patient was almost a quarter of a million dollars. Back in 1984 Dr. Herbert Baum, director of Data and Research Services, Elm Services, Inc., Rockville, Maryland, estimated the lifetime loss to be $416,500. On a national scale the annual loss for the MS population as a whole was estimated to be $1.6 billion. Today that figure would be even higher.

These facts and figures are, frankly, intolerable. In addition to the financial impact, think of the loss of contributions made by the MS population. There could be a Jonas Salk, a Hemingway, an Iacocca in the ranks of the MS population.

What can you do? Get tough. Strengthen your will. And, possibly, get a lawyer. But first, get in a mind-set that no one, no disease, or no discriminatory attitude is going to stand in your way. Focus on one career goal at a time and go for it. If you have many goals, make a list of your priorities. Then, starting with number one, list all the things that could make you more successful in achieving that goal.

First and foremost, there must be a motivation. Not everyone has the same ambitions. But whatever you're going to be, you still have the right to work, maintain your dignity, and not give up. This must be the generation of trailblazers. It's your obligation to try to stay in the work force and get those statistics up.

With an MS diagnosis you're likely to take a hard look at your career. It's sort of what happens to people when they turn fifty and take stock of what their lives mean. The only difference is that you may be twenty-eight, and it's a little early for such lofty reflection. Still, you may realize that you've been stuck in a dead-end job for the past few years anyway, and if you've ever thought of taking a risk, you should do it now in the event that you're not healthy enough to take it later. Or you may decide to finish that advanced degree. Often, with age on your side, and in an early stage, an MS diagnosis may spur you on to actually do things you might never have done otherwise. The person with a slightly more advanced form of MS may go through the same emotional reaction but may not choose to act so impulsively. How do you know how to plan your life and when to act on those plans? The unpredictability factor makes this really tough. Talk to a few friends, one devil-may-care, another conservative. Listen to different viewpoints and process the advice given. Finally, look at the benefits package where you're working. What will happen to your insurance, your pension? Do they offer a disability package? You don't have to throw your dreams out the window, but if you're the sole supporter of a family, for instance, you might opt for the more conservative choice. But be creative. You might decide to stay with the company and start a new business venture on the side.

MS and Your Present Job

Should you tell your boss and co-workers about your MS? That really depends on your length of time with the company, your preexisting relationships, and the office politics and competition. If your MS is invisible, we suggest keeping the diagnosis to yourself. Those three people waiting to move into your job might just "sympathetically" discuss how your illness is affecting your job even when it isn't. "She really looks tired lately" is something that could be said about anyone.

If signs and symptoms have been visible and there is knowledge that you have undergone diagnostic tests, you may choose to inform your immediate boss or the superior with whom you have the best rapport. The disclosure may be better than the suspicion that your wobbly walk was due to a three-martini lunch. Probably, you will already have proved your on-the-job performance and your contribution to the company. If this is the case, reinforce your attributes and express a desire to continue. If you were on shaky ground on the job before your MS, don't expect anyone to feel sorry for you and keep you on in spite of your inadequacy. Assess your skills carefully. Maybe you need to make a lateral shift into a job that you can do better.

Stay in optimal mental health. Studies show that many sick days for the whole work population are really mental health days, hangover days, and the like. From time to time, you are going to need sick days for MS, so make sure you cut out all other absentee days. You can no longer afford that luxury. You've got to show you're a reliable employee.

MS and a Prospective Employer

Job hunting for the person with MS is a whole different ball game. You're going to have to sell yourself and compete with many other job applicants. The only way you are going to win that job is if you think like a winner. This is easier said than done when the cloud of MS hangs clearly on the horizon. For your job interview, at least, you are going to have to rid yourself of negative thoughts and fears. First, you must be fully prepared for the interview. Do research about the company. How long has it been in business? What do you know about its competition? Develop strong reasons why you'd like to work for the company other than you have MS and you could really use a job. It may very well be your primary reason, but by no means tell that to a prospective employer. In fact, if you really concentrate on the other reasons for seeking a particular job, you might succeed in taking even subconscious thoughts of MS out of the job interview.

Do not go into an interview prepared for rejection. Visualize that you are going to shake on the deal. If someone else gets the job, you'll deal with the disappointment later. But right now, psych yourself up and go in on top of the world. One woman actually plays the theme song from *Rocky* while getting dressed for job interviews. She also calls her best friend on the phone and they go through an uplifting ritual together. Assuming the role of a fight manager, the friend repeats over and over, "Remember, you're the best. You're the champ. You're gonna win this one." They often burst out laughing at points in the ritual, but it still puts all the right positive forces to work.

Tips for Those with Visible Symptoms

If you have visible symptoms, you are going to have to address your situation up front. People, no matter how worldly, intelligent, or sophisticated, often feel uncomfortable around people with disabilities. There is only one way to make them feel comfortable and that is to be comfortable with yourself. If you use a cane or a wheelchair, you might prefer to break the ice on the telephone when you are setting up the interview. After you set up the time and the date, drop this information in almost as an afterthought. "Oh, one other thing. I have a temporary (or slight) disability, so I'd just like to make sure I can arrange for convenient parking. Where would you suggest?"

Don't talk about MS unless the interviewer brings it up. If you are asked about your disability, answer without hesitation. Either say you have MS or something more vague, such as that you're recovering from an "old neurological problem." It's good to add, whether it's true at the moment or not, that you're feeling terrific. Never complain to people with whom you may work.

Rehearse these questions and answers with your mate or a friend or job counselor. Have them role-play the job interviewer and go over every imaginable question. Find what answers feel right for you. And learn to be a bit of an actor. That's what Ronald Reagan did before each presidential debate with Walter Mondale. His aides grilled and drilled him and threw him every possible left hook In fact, he didn't do so well in the first debate at all, seeming slow and too old.

He dropped a few points in the polls, and it seemed he was on shaky ground. But Reagan was a fighter. He analyzed his weaknesses and came back for the next debate. He was not going to let his age be a hindrance, so he dispelled the issue before it became one. With poise and humor, Ronald Reagan charmed his way into his second presidency, despite the critical issue of his age. If you, too, prepare intensely for your interviews, then visualize getting the job, you can get the job you want. You may blow an interview or two, but remember what happened to Reagan in his first debate.

You may choose, for instance, to address the issue of absenteeism. Tell the interviewer that it will probably be less than other employees, since you are more sensitive to company concerns than the average person. Don't sound or act defensive, but if you sense the employer may still have doubts, be creative. Volunteer to use your vacation days in the event you have more sick days than you anticipate. But again, spend as little time as possible discussing MS. Move on to other interview areas quickly and with confidence. With some experience, you will learn how to change the subject politely. One way is to ask if you may ask some questions. Play it by ear. If you have sensed that the interviewer likes a go-getter type, inquire about company policy on internal mobility. Say, for instance, that while you're certain you'll be very satisfied with the job available, you are still curious about growth opportunities.

With or without MS, good jobs are hard to get. Don't get discouraged if an interview doesn't go well. Go home and analyze what went right and what went wrong. You'll get better and better with practice. Be tough on yourself. You need that winning edge to nail the job next time. Just don't be defeatist in the process. After all, you'll never know if the real reason you were turned down for the job was that the boss had to hire his wife's nephew.

If you are having difficulty figuring out where you fit in the work force, some chapters of the National MS Society offer a "Job Raising" program that gives career guidance, résumé counseling, and more.

In conclusion, if your MS is invisible, we do not advise disclosing it while job hunting. Too many people have experienced rejection, placement in dead-end jobs, or early dismissal. Get the job, prove yourself, become a star performer or a good solid worker, and then disclose your MS if you really want to. But, just as in other relationships, first ask yourself why you have a need to tell someone.

If disclosing your MS on the job or in the job interview is necessary for obvious reasons, mention it, but don't make it the focus of your career. Emphasize that you are a hard worker and that you know you can contribute greatly to the company. While you can't blame every career problem on MS, be aware of discrimination. If a prospective employer tells you outright that you're qualified but that he doesn't think a person with a disability would work out too well in the job, you may have legal recourse. After the interview write down your recollections of the conversation as accurately as possible. You may need them later.

Discrimination doesn't only happen in such overt ways. Perhaps you've been passed over for a promotion just because of your boss's prejudice or lack of comfort with your MS. This is tricky—many people think it's better to hang on to a job than kick up the dust because they don't have a better one. Not everyone is cut out to be a crusader, but not everyone should just take it on the chin, either. It's a fact of life that MS sometimes shortens careers. Fatigue and cognitive impairment are often the cause. But it is unacceptable to let discrimination do it first.

Since 1992, the American Disabilities Act has protected people in the workplace from discrimination. The ADA has a definition of "disability" that each person must meet: you must have a physical or mental impairment that limits one or more major life activities and medical records of that impairment. Some people with MS do not qualify. Many will. Any company with fifteen or more employees must accommodate disability in the workplace. But it's up to you to request what is needed.

Accommodations about which you might ask include moving your workstation closer to the restroom; access to a refrigerator; a work space with cooler temperature; flexible work hours or occasional work from home; reduction of physical exertion; an ergonomic workstation; reduction in walking; grab bars in the rest rooms, and more. If your employer resists helping you perform your job with a disability, he or she may be in violation of the law.

If you haven't disclosed your MS to your employer, you might begin with a doctor's letter describing accommodation you need because of a neurological impairment. But understand that ultimately, under law, your employer does not have to comply without a more specific diagnosis. Weigh your personal situation, both financial and emotional, and decide if you can afford to take action. In the meantime, you, too, should keep accurate notes of your work experience and contributions. Be realistic about your performance. Was the promotion promised to you before you had MS? Were you told you were being groomed for the position? Are your colleagues shocked at the ultimate decision? Then it's up to you whether or not to consult an attorney or the American Civil Liberties Union. If you do want to see an attorney, ask your neurologist or local bar association for a lawyer with a specialty in the area. And when you call the attorney to make an appointment, make sure you ask whether or not there is a consultation fee for the initial visit.

10

If the Person with MS Is Someone You Care About

Multiple sclerosis strikes about two hundred people a week in addition to the more than a quarter of a million who have already been diagnosed as having the disease. But MS affects millions more. For every one person who lives with the disease, there is an "extended family" that will also be greatly impacted. Just because MS isn't in your central nervous system doesn't mean it's not in your life. Whether the person with MS is your spouse, your lover, your parent, your child, or your good friend, if you care about someone with MS, you've earned a seat on the same roller coaster. You've probably already felt panicked, helpless, guilty, heartbroken, frustrated, fearful, and more. Well, fasten your seat belt. Although there are no magical solutions to all of your problems, we have plenty of suggestions to make the ride a lot less bumpy.

MS is a disease that brings with it times of crisis. Relationships can either be strained, strengthened, or both. But it's important to realize that MS never ruins relationships—only people do. And no matter how well the person with MS is coping, it takes two to maintain the bonds of a relationship.

The person with MS must sharpen his or her emotional skills, but so must the person close by. While the damage MS inflicts on the central nervous system is beyond your control, the damage it inflicts on your relationship isn't.

How relationships are affected is determined both by the personalities of those involved and by the individual case of MS. It would be impossible to discuss every potential relationship problem at every stage of every type of MS. We have therefore selected the universal issues. Some may be more relevant to milder cases, while others may only concern those with more severe disability. You'll know which sections apply to your situation.

Disclosure

Your involvement with MS begins with the disclosure that your loved one has it. The disclosure may be either at the same time the patient finds out or later, when the person with MS chooses to tell you.

When you learn of the diagnosis at the same time as your loved one, you will most likely experience the same emotional phases—shock, denial, anger, and eventual acceptance—we discussed in chapter 8. It is unlikely that two people will enter each phase at the same time, but often one will pull the other through. One person may feel shock longer; the other may get angrier faster. There is no timetable to follow; it will just have to take its natural course. But since your adjustment may be beginning now, we'll walk you through the stages of getting there. Not only do you want to understand what you're feeling, you also hope to do everything you can for your loved one.

At the time of diagnosis, the MS patient will make a conscious or unconscious choice of whom to lean on. Be sensitive to the choice. It may not be you. If you are not the spouse, for example, but someone very close just the same, make sure you're not interfering in the dynamics of what the couple must go through together. Or if you know the patient's big brother has always been able to work magic, give them some room. See who's around, and try to figure out where you best fit in. Be sensitive but be there. If you've been informed, you've been involved. Listen, give support and reassurance, but don't give advice. The diagnosis is no time to discuss job changes or moving into a one-story house. If this is your first experience with MS, you'll need a crash information course before you do anything more than offer comfort. Even if you've read a lot of material, it's going to take time to absorb the information and process how it fits into everyone's life.

There will be plenty of time to deal with important issues down the road. First, deal with the shock and grieving period that follow a diagnosis. Most important, help get the person with MS through the current episode. If an exacerbation is still in progress, make sure the patient is following doctor's orders. If the newly diagnosed person is in a denial phase, he or she may, for instance, refuse to take prescribed medications or refuse to rest. Don't assume someone else is monitoring the situation. Check it out yourself. If there is a problem, don't talk to the person like a child who won't swallow the cough syrup. Address the person in a straightforward manner and say, "At the risk of sounding like an armchair psychologist, I think this is what you're doing. . . ."

Unless the doctor has ordered otherwise, extend regular invitations to get out of the house. If you always go out for Sunday brunch, try to keep the routine going. It's okay to try a little coaching if your invitation is declined, but don't push too hard. Understand that emotional healing is in progress, and some people prefer to stay inside the home. When this happens, put yourself on call for when the person is ready to go out and get some fresh air.

When disclosure of your loved one's MS comes later, there is a different set of emotions to deal with. The person with MS has already gone through the initial emotional stages and has begun to come to terms with it. By the time the disclosure is made to you, the person with MS is ready to talk about it with you. Feel free to ask questions. If it is a well-thought-out disclosure, the person with MS has chosen a moment of strength to tell you and is emotionally prepared to face your reaction. Keep the dialogue going as long as you both need to.

Because you are very close to that person, you may be offended or angry that you weren't informed sooner. A lover might feel betrayed because the relationship was allowed to flourish without such an important disclosure. A parent might be hurt by being left out and at a loss as to why his or her nurturing skills weren't called on. One friend might be furious that another friend knew all this time and she didn't. Maybe these are valid emotions, but maybe they're not. Sometimes, when fielding a big emotional curveball like MS, our emotions get displaced. Think of the family funeral at which there's a big fuss over someone who said the wrong thing or wore the wrong color dress. The poor soul, who was just trying to pay respect, becomes the object of bitter conversation for what seems like hours. Is the family really angry at that person? Not at all. Their pain over the death is so profound that it's easier to get angry over the color of a dress than it is to tap their real grief of the moment. Similar emotional turmoil can follow an MS disclosure by a loved one. If you understand it, you can avoid it.

Instead of getting angry that you weren't told sooner, ask yourself why you were told now. Does the person need your help or support at the moment? Was he or she trying to protect you before? Has your life situation changed so that he or she feels the timing is more appropriate for you now? Did the person need time to deal with it alone before involving you?

Has your relationship bonded into something more meaningful than before? Was he or she afraid of rejection? There are many answers to "why now?" The odds are that the one you'll hear will at least be understandable.

Finally, if you think about it, you should take comfort in the fact that you had no idea your loved one had MS. This means that the disability is not visible and he or she has chosen not to make MS the focus of life. You now share a private secret. Learn about it, talk about it, but don't dwell on it.

EDUCATION

After the disclosure, the next step is getting good information about MS. The National MS Society is a very good source, but it's not in the publishing business. The lack of honest, accurate, and helpful information is our motivation for writing this book. MS is a disease with many different courses and many different phases. Much of the literature lumps all MS problems together without making the necessary distinctions. A book with an entire chapter dedicated to bladder problems may lead you to believe this is a chronic problem for everyone with MS, even though it's not. For a minority of people with untreated infections, it can be life-threatening, and perhaps this is the rationale for the emphasis. But, for the person learning about MS for the first time, the message can be frightening. Also, don't read old literature. Recent advances paint a whole new picture. Beware of subliminal messages. These are subconscious thoughts that register without your realizing it. For instance, in the library you may find books on MS with pictures of wheelchairs on the cover, a truly unfortunate choice by some publisher who ignored the fact that the majority of MS patients will never need wheelchairs.

Feature articles and personal anecdotes are no better. Some are honest and enlightening, such as Moira K. Griffin's "The Courage Not to Fall Apart" in *Self* magazine (January 1986). In the article, Griffin, an avid runner, writes poignantly:

> *Frankly, it's hard not to resent it when some women run by me now, and I think they're only trying to trim their thighs, while it takes blood, sweat and tears just to make mine work. But I also know I'm lucky that my thighs work as well as they do. Of course, this may not last. There's only one predictable thing about MS, and that's that it's unpredictable. Maybe someday I won't be able to run. But right now I can, so I will—with joy.*

This introspective article, however, is the exception rather then the rule. Unfortunately, editors find only the bleakest stories to be "inspirational." One that comes to mind is about a woman who, despite her horrible condition, had learned to communicate with her children through blinking. Such cases are so incredibly rare that it's a good idea to avoid such literature. While we think it's vital to learn the facts about MS, it serves no purpose to read about every depressing textbook tragedy. If you wanted to read about the flu, would you look for an article about people who die from it? Of course not. You'd want to know what happens to most people who get it and what you can do to get over it. Do the same with MS.

You might also be drawn to television or film accounts of MS. Keep in mind that movies such as the ten-hankie *Duet for One* (first a successful Broadway play) are made for theatrical impact, not educational purposes. After all, tragedy is the stuff of which great drama is made. William Shakespeare didn't write *Romeo and Juliet* with a happy ending. And *Wuthering Heights* would never have had the same impact if

Heathcliff hadn't had to carry his true love to the window as she lay dying in his arms.

Tugging at your heartstrings applies to some MS fund-raisers and public service announcements as well. Will the National MS Society raise more money if it presents a successful career woman with invisible MS in long-term remission or a young adult in a wheelchair?

If your loved one has a history of remissions or is in remission at the present time, don't let these media images stick in your mind. Don't be an ostrich and stick your head in the sand, either, but find a way to distance yourself. Deal only with the situation at hand, and believe that the person in your life who has MS has a very good chance of having a mild course or at least one for which there are excellent treatments. You don't want to paint a tragedy that may never happen to you.

What's in a Name?

It's a good idea to get comfortable with the words *multiple sclerosis* and MS so that you can talk about it more easily with someone who has it. Although it never happened before, somehow now that MS has touched your life, the words seem to get caught in your throat on the way out of your mouth. Although you may prefer to use phrases that are less direct, such as *this problem* or *your illness,* get over it. Dancing around the terminology is a signal that you're dancing around the real issues at hand. If this is a problem, try a technique used in sex therapy. When people are uncomfortable verbalizing words like *penis* or *vagina,* they are coached to repeat the word over and over until it's no big deal to say it anymore. Doing this with the words *multiple sclerosis* will help get you over this first hurdle of communication. After all, how can you solve a problem you can't talk about?

While on the subject of language, you may or may not have noticed that throughout the book, we usually make references to *people with MS* or *people with multiple sclerosis.* We don't use other common terms such as *MSer, MS victim, handicapped, differently abled, physically challenged,* or *crippled.* We don't even use the term *MS patient* unless it is in the context of being diagnosed, treated, or counseled by a physician. We strongly favor a choice of language that avoids both negative and patronizing undertones. Our choice, we believe, allows for the greatest degree of dignity, reinforcing the message that those who get this disease are ordinary people who have a specific medical problem.

Others may have different choices, so why not ask? You have to make *them* happy, not us. In her book, *Plain Text,* Nancy Mairs explains that she actually prefers the word *cripple.* She wants people to know the difficulties she faces. For her, *cripple* is an educated social statement. For most people, however, it can be a serious social slur.

Denial: The Most Vicious Enemy

One of the most common and serious emotional affronts to the person with MS is denial by those who are close. Especially when symptoms are invisible, it's hard to believe the person with MS is sick at all. In therapy groups from coast to coast, the same story is heard over and over. The person with MS just looks too damn good for others to believe he or she has a disease that sounds so foreboding. Although anyone can get stuck in the denial phase, more anecdotes seem to be relayed about husbands who never seem to accept that anything is wrong. Some of these denials are incredibly blatant—the husband even refuses to believe the diagnosis coming straight from the doctor's mouth. Other denials are more subtle. A diagnosis might be accepted, but real complaints are written off as either insignificant or due to other causes.

Beyond that, there can be a refusal to discuss MS at all. Even when the person with MS experiences a long period of remission, the subject is going to come up. A current news report on a research discovery, the decision to make a year-end charitable contribution to the National MS Society—whatever the reason, the subject is going to come up from time to time. Don't fall into the trap of not wanting to hear about it. If a certified neurologist has given your loved one a definite MS diagnosis, you've got to believe it. Don't fool yourself that this is some kind of mistake. Denial on the part of another is one of the most painful things a person with MS has to deal with. The alienation it causes can be devastating.

This must be distinguished from "healthy denial," in which you are helping your loved one make MS less of a focus in life. An unhealthy denial is when you're convinced the person with MS is just fine. Do you refuse discussion of MS? Have you refused all suggestions to attend therapy sessions or support groups? Do you find yourself minimizing complaints or creating other reasons for symptoms? Have you ever found yourself saying something like, "Oh, it's not fatigue. You're just down in the dumps. Get out of the house for a while, you'll feel a lot better"? Has someone handed you this book with this page earmarked? Don't be stubborn. Make an appointment and talk to the neurologist or counselor on your own. Take down the walls and enrich your relationship. The consequences of denial can be severe.

Advice for the Spouse

When the person with MS is your spouse, it is quite normal to feel a spectrum of emotions you may be too embarrassed or guilty to admit. Although you, too, vowed to love, honor, and cherish in sickness and in health, you never expected to be put to the test so soon. Now you're worrying if your own life will be dragged down, if your career will be held back, if you'll wind up trapped, burdened, and financially drained. And what's worse, you also feel you should be shot for even letting such selfish thoughts cross your mind. Don't beat yourself up. While you can't only think of "me, me, me," you're certainly entitled to wonder how this is going to affect your personal life. Any extraordinary circumstance such as a chronic illness will trigger such a reaction.

If you've read this book from the beginning to this page, you've already learned that the majority of people with MS have periods of remission, often years at a time, with a return to normal or near normal after each attack. But you've also learned there are no guarantees. Regardless of how educated about the disease you are, the unpredictability of MS can still get to you. It's true that you don't know what's down the road in five or ten years. You also don't know what's down the road for your own health picture in that time period. You may fantasize about another relationship or wish you were married to someone else. That's normal. Right now your partner is wishing he or she could make a trade for another body, too. Think about anything you like. But don't run off and have an affair. Tough this situation out without adding a "triangle" to your problems. And think about this. If you found a new partner, could you be sure he or she would remain the picture of health? No one has any guarantees. (One in four people will get cancer. We'll skip the laundry list of everything else that can happen.)

Having MS isn't a good reason to bail out of a relationship. It's simply something to work around. Think of MS like a mother-in-law. She's there, but you're not going to let her interfere in your marriage. Your financial picture may change, your roles may change, but that could have happened under many other circumstances, too. Your marriage will survive a lot of self-imposed limitations. But it won't survive without romance and shared experiences. Right now, be flexible, and reignite the romance in your marriage. Your mate may be depressed or frustrated by MS. Or he or she may be so fearful that your marriage won't survive that he or she is acting withdrawn or self-protective. Don't let these fears become self-fulfilling prophecies. Plan a romantic evening. Take the television set out of the bedroom. Try out a new body massage cream. Throw out your old ratty bathrobes and bring home sexy new ones for both of you. Or check into a motel for the night. Just have fun together. And remind your partner that you can lose the car, you can lose the house, you can lose just about anything, but you can't lose your sense of humor.

The couple that stops playing together won't be staying together very long. If skiing is the great passion of your life and MS doesn't allow your partner to join you on the slopes anymore, figure out a solution. You can still go to the resort together, and your partner can enjoy snowmobiling or other activities, or perhaps you'll take a quickie ski trip on your own. Talk out all the pros and cons and be honest. If you're not, you run the risk that one or both of you will harbor resentment. Approach each compromise as an experiment. Don't feel that the success or failure of your marriage hangs in the balance with each project. But do compromise. If, for instance, you stubbornly insist that you're going dirt biking every weekend, even though your partner can no longer enjoy such a strenuous activity, he or she isn't going to mope about your selfishness forever. In adjusting to MS, he or she is going to find new recreational activities and new people with whom to enjoy them. No one is asking you to give up your favorite sport. We're just reminding you that you can't leave someone in (or out of) the dust every single weekend. Just because a person has MS doesn't mean he or she is going to take second-class treatment. Dig down deep inside for the root of your selfishness. Are you really a louse or are you actually running away from the realities at home? Don't be a coward. The reality at home isn't nearly as bad as the situation you're creating by dodging it. Don't take the easy way out. Stick around, and find new wonderful things you'll love doing together. You don't have to give up dirt biking completely or forever. It's unlikely to be the only hobby in the world you enjoy so much—it's probably the *first* hobby you discovered you enjoy that much.

Advice for Parents

MS usually strikes at an age when a parent's active child rearing is over. The parent-child roles have been redefined for better or for worse. You, the parent, may finally have begun to enjoy a part of life with less responsibility. With college bills out of the way, you'd been thinking more toward your retirement fund and personal desires. But your adult child's MS diagnosis has thrown you for a loop. You were hoping your child would look after you in your sunset years. Now that looks like it's in jeopardy, too. What's more, your instinct is to jump in and make it all better, but your parental guidance may not even be wanted right now.

Hang on and take one step at a time. Everyone wants to remain independent, and it is to be hoped that everyone can. You, too, are going to have to learn to take one step at a time and not go crazy worrying about all the "what ifs." You've done a proper job in preparing your child to face adversity. However, no one is expected to be ready to face an incurable illness, so don't analyze what you did right and what you did wrong.

As you learn about the disease, you may wonder if it's something you passed along to your child. Parents wind up feeling guilty about everything. You've probably read that although MS is not a hereditary disease, there is a "genetic susceptibility" that can run in a family. Don't beat yourself up over this, either. Scientists also believe exposure to an as-yet-undiscovered virus before age fifteen may be what causes genetically susceptible people to develop MS. No parent is expected to raise a child in a bubble. It's not your fault, so don't act as if it is. It's something that just happens.

Often a parent is the most devastated when something happens to a child. This can be an extra burden on the person with MS. Not only does that person feel rotten about having the disease, he or she now has to worry about the trauma of the parent. Don't let this get out of hand. If you're having trouble coping, either get tough or get help. If you're the emotional type, you can cry, throw your own dishes, and go through your own grieving period, but you're going to have to get your act together sometime. If you don't, you're bound to smother your child when he or she would rather have an extra friend.

Occasionally an adult child will regress and become psychologically dependent on the parent. The person with MS can actually revert to behavior patterns from childhood. Independence, not regression, should be encouraged by the parent. If the problem is severe, professional help should be suggested.

A parent of a child with MS might want to reassess life insurance policies and wills. Depending on the individual situation and the status of other family members, you may choose new estate planning. Discuss this with your child and your lawyer or financial adviser. Whether through discrimination, the high divorce rate, or actual job-related disability, MS will unfortunately cut the lifetime earnings of many, probably most, people who have it. If you want to do something constructive, make the necessary accommodations for the person with MS in your will.

An MS diagnosis, like any crisis, tends to put other things in perspective. Although it's not the time to rehash old problems, it is the time to repair unresolved emotions in a family. The adult child who's always felt like the family disappointment, for instance, is going to feel worse. It may be time to sit down and say the things you never said before. Trace back through the moments you felt proud of your child but for whatever reason never said anything. Now is the time to focus on "personal bests." There's no more comparing your child to other children, neighbors, or cousins. Did he or she achieve a personal best? Reflect on it, and think about how you can help or encourage your adult child to reach one now. Don't help your adult child set unrealistic goals—either too high or too low. You're going to have to find the right balance for yourselves. Be ready to have some anger coming your way; it's all part of what happens as the dust settles.

If your adult child learns to make MS less and less a focus of life, you have to also. One well-adjusted account executive blurted out at the dinner table one day that the only time she thought about her MS was when her mother brought it up. This, unfortunately, was constantly. The well-meaning mom was actually a pain in the neck and the only obstacle in the way of a totally adjusted existence.

On the other hand, don't avoid subjects just because you think they are painful. A father shouldn't avoid talking with his son about dating or sex just because the son has MS. Those mother-daughter talks shouldn't come to a halt either. The adult child with MS wants more than anything for you to go back to acting like a normal parent.

Ultimately, your adult child will let you know if you help or add to the problem. If your adult child is seeing less and less of everyone, there is a bigger problem than you. But if he or she has healthy relationships with others and seems alienated toward you, there's a good chance it's something you do that doesn't feel very comforting. It might be something you're unaware of, like a look of pity or fear in your eye. Or you might be trying too hard, joking inappropriately, or acting very clingy. If you can't figure it out, ask what it is. Your child might not even know exactly. But talk. Remind your child that you're doing the best you can, too, and that you're willing to try a little harder. If it's the only way to get your child to open up, be provocative. Listen closely, don't get defensive, and make sure you're not getting a bad rap. You might find out it's not your fault at all, that underneath it all, he or she is rebelling against the idea of feeling dependent on you. Make the necessary repairs. You'll get through this a lot easier together.

ADVICE FOR LOVERS

Advice really isn't necessary for the casual lover of a person with MS. All you really need is a reminder that it's not contagious. Casual love affairs are fine, but by their very nature include no acceptance of emotional responsibility. Advice for a lover with more serious intentions is far more difficult. Unlike a spouse, you have not taken a vow to love, honor, and cherish in sickness and in health, and you have no long-term commitment or obligation. You just happen to be in love, and learning that he or she has MS has thrown you completely for a loop. After all, throughout this heart-thumping phase in your relationship, you've been convinced you've met the most wonderful, perfect person ever. You love the way that person talks and the way that person smells. Everything he or she says is insightful and clever. Things that will bug the hell out of you ten years down the line right now are perfectly adorable. And the best thing is, no one has ever understood all your complexities this clearly. Now there's MS and the shock that this perfect person really isn't perfect. In fact, the person you're in love with has an incurable disease.

Although all the people indirectly involved with MS have many emotional issues in common, you have one issue to face all on your own. You have to decide if you can deal with getting married or you have to deal with the decision that you can't. Some painful soul-searching is going to be required as the meaning of "for better or for worse" becomes much more real. No one will be able to give you any answers. Some may be able to accept this news but others may not. If you are the type of personality who tends to be overly fearful of what the future may hold or you are a "worrier" type, this problem may bring out the worst side of you. Take your time in thinking out your decision. Ask your partner's permission to consult with the neurologist and set up an appointment. (Permission is necessary to breach patient-doctor confidentiality.) Then talk to your lover and try to sort out, with tenderness, how you both feel. This is a moment for great strength and bravery on both your parts. Underneath is a great love affair that feels like it's crumbling. It is not. You both still love each other. That doesn't change. The decision to stay together forever, however, just might.

Interestingly, couples who do ultimately choose to stay together have a great chance of a successful marriage. The strength of their love for each other is tested before they exchange their vows, and they pass with flying colors. It is not uncommon to live "happily ever after" in spite of MS. Not everyone makes that choice, however, and if you choose not to make a commitment to someone with MS, that is your prerogative. You must, however, be honest. There is no other reason you can invent that will be believable. It will probably make you feel better if you wait a "grace" period and then find some other reason to break up, but this is deceitful and more painful. If you determine you do not want to remain with someone who has MS, you must identify the reason and explain it lovingly. In the words of the Seven Sages, "Know thyself." Then once you do, you must reveal to your partner that you are too fearful, too selfish, too inflexible, and so on. Explain that you both should move on because although you are in love, you are no longer compatible for the long haul. Then move on. Don't drag things out and suggest compromises like, "We should try seeing other people." You are mature people who are in love and if you chose to cut the cord, you must.

If you find this notion unacceptable, then you must rethink your decision. Maybe you aren't giving yourself enough credit, or maybe the situation isn't as bleak as it appeared at first. Don't think of what your friends would do, and don't think of what your families will have to say about your decision. The decision is yours and yours alone. They will not live with this situation, only you will. They do not understand the depth of your love or the depth of your fear. If you are thinking of others' opinions, you are not mature enough to make this decision. Ultimately, if you find yourself too confused to make any decision, seek professional guidance from a therapist or member of the clergy who can give you premarriage counseling.

In conclusion, when you learn someone you love has MS, it is not the end of the world nor is it the end of your relationship. With maturity, common sense, and love, relationships can flourish and even become stronger. It's up to both of you.

11

New Hope for a Cure

Now that you know what MS is, how you treat the symptoms, and how you can best cope with it, there is one more great pressing question—"How close is the cure?" As we'll explain in this chapter, it's right around the corner.

This is not meant to build up false hopes. We say the cure is right around the corner with one strong qualification best summed up by Dr. Stephen Reingold, now retired but for many years, head of research and director of grants management for the National Multiple Sclerosis Society in New York. He explained:

> *The answer depends on something significant—that everything we've learned so far is in the right direction. This is not a criticism of MS research, in particular, it is an inherent problem with research in general. When you deal with a mystery, you follow clues and you develop strategies. You go down paths and make decisions at certain points based on the evidence that you've accumulated. The beauty of the scientific process is that if you're doing it right, those paths will lead you to an ultimate conclusion or answer to the question that you're asking. But there's always the*

> *possibility that as you go around the bend, you're going to be struck by something that you hadn't thought of before which will set you back twenty steps.*

Ever since MS was first defined as a disease, some doctor has claimed the cure is near. We know that people have been misled every decade because of premature claims. But the truth is that today, scientific evidence has reached such a sophisticated level that we truly believe the cause of MS will soon be proved and this will rapidly lead to a real cure.

Scientists today are working on the premise that MS is an autoimmune system disease triggered by a virus. The way to tell whether something is an autoimmune disease or not is to take an animal with the disease, remove immune system cells, transfer them to a new animal without the disease, and see if the new animal gets the disease. If it does, it proves the disease is autoimmune. In MS studies of guinea pigs, rats, and mice, this has been proved, although here we must add another slight qualification. Because they don't know how it is contracted, scientists are not able to give MS to animals. All laboratory animal tests use a disease that is very similar to MS, *experimental allergic encephalomyelitis (EAE)*. It is the closest disease to MS that scientists have to work with, but it is not exactly MS.

EAE became the animal model for MS through a long process. EAE actually developed as a result of complications associated with the Pasteur antirabies vaccine in the 1890s. At that time some people were found to be "hypersensitive" to the Pasteur antirabies vaccine and developed paralysis—an unexpected reaction to the vaccine, which was made from rabbit myelin. In hypersensitive people, the foreign myelin stimulated the immune system to put out anti-myelin antibodies that then attached to the myelin in the human brain and caused damage. This was the first evidence of a myelin disease due to an autoimmune reaction.

In 1933 scientists discovered that by injecting normal brain tissue into monkeys over a period of time, they could produce an experimental demyelinating disease in the laboratory. In the 1940s scientists searching for a more practical animal model further refined EAE with the addition of an *adjuvant*—certain oils and bacterial cells that shortened the production of the disease from months to weeks. EAE could now be made by taking myelin from one monkey, mixing it with the adjuvant, and injecting it into the foot pad of another monkey. Within about eight days, the second monkey would get a neurological disease that had many signs of human MS and showed myelin damage in the brain and spinal cord. At that time scientists also learned how to produce the disease in other animal species. This new animal model for MS was a real boon to research except for one distinguishing characteristic—EAE was a one-time only disease, while MS is predominantly relapsing. It wasn't until 1983 that researchers were able to refine a chronic-relapsing EAE (strain 13) in guinea pigs. This is the closest laboratory model ever to MS. It fulfills four important criteria necessary to make it a laboratory *analog* for MS:

1. Delayed onset.
2. Chronic-progressive or -relapsing course.
3. Large plaques with demyelination associated with inflammation.
4. Widespread distribution of plaques.

While scientists continue to try to perfect EAE, it is a very good animal model for research.

The two most important questions being asked in MS research today are, What is really wrong with the immune system? and, What is the foreign body, or *antigen* it is responding to?

The immune system is the body's protection against invasion of antigens such as bacteria, viruses, pollen, additives, certain foods, and others. When a person is first introduced to an antigen, such as a flu virus, the immune system makes an *antibody,* or protective chemical, to fight off the invader. The next time the person is exposed to the same flu virus, the immune system remembers, recognizes the invader, and releases the specific antibodies that react with the virus and destroy it. Incredibly, the immune system can produce antibodies with the identical shape of the antigen they must bind with point for point in order to eliminate the antigen, allowing the person to recover. Antibodies are made by white blood cells called *lymphocytes,* which originate in bone marrow and circulate through the bloodstream, patrolling all areas of the body to identify and protect against foreign invaders. When the lymph nodes in the body swell, it's actually because they're filling up with these cells which will attack the invader.

Today, through state-of-the-art biotechnology, scientists can now identify two basic types of lymphocytes called *B cells* and *T cells.* The B cells produce antibodies that neutralize certain components of invaders (such as in chicken pox or mumps). The T cells act more directly to kill foreign invaders. Some are *cytotoxic cells,* which punch holes in the antigen. Others are *T-helper cells,* which enhance the role of other immune system cells and can activate the *macrophages,* which eat every foreign invader in their path, almost like a Pac Man gobbling up debris. Secretions from the T-helper cells also activate *natural killer (NK) cells,* which play an important but not yet fully understood role in fighting viral infections. Finally, there are *T-suppressor cells* which turn off the immune system response once the invader is completely destroyed.

The immune system, made up of many subsets of B and

T cells, is a very carefully regulated system. Besides the interaction between lymphocytes, macrophages, and antibodies, the immune system also recognizes *self* or *nonself*. In other words, it can tell the difference between your own liver and a transplanted one. It will know that the new liver is not the one that should be there, genetically, and it will reject it unless the immune system is toned down through such immunosuppressant drugs as cyclosporine.

Some scientists believe MS may be caused by a lack of recognition of self versus nonself. It is possible that the immune system registers myelin as an antigen to attack. This is supported by the knowledge that B cells, T cells, and macrophages accumulate at the lesion site in MS. What actually causes the myelin damage is still under investigation. Some researchers believe the T cells latch onto myelin and activate the macrophages, which then attack and eat the myelin. Others believe that B lymphocytes make antibodies that bind to myelin and guide macrophages to the target. Perhaps two or more events are happening simultaneously in MS.

Besides lack of recognition, it is also possible that MS is caused by a "screw-up" in the regulation of the immune system—that a helper-inducer subset of immune system cells, which help keep the immune response going, is numerically or functionally overrepresented. Or suppressor-inducer cells, which might tone down immune response, may be numerically or functionally underrepresented in MS.

A study reported in January 1987 by Dr. Howard L. Weiner, co-director of the Center for Neurologic Diseases at Harvard Medical School, showed that the suppressor cells are indeed underrepresented, at least in patients with progressive MS. Weiner discovered the patients had only about half the normal level of the subset T-4 suppressor-inducer cell.

In October 1989 British researchers reported that EAE was, indeed, related to "bad T-cells."

Today, researchers have identified a new T cell, called *T regs*, which are different from the white blood cells believed to cause the attack in MS. T regs are now being researched to see if they actually inhibit the immune response. A small study at Harvard's Brigham and Women's Hospital in Boston in 2004 compared T reg cells of 15 people with remitting-relapsing MS to the T regs of 21 people without MS. Although the T reg cell count was the same in each group, the T regs were significantly impaired in the group with MS.

A 2005 study of mice with EAE showed researchers could alter the course of disease progress by helping impaired T reg cells function.

One treatment currently under investigation for people with relapsing and progressive MS is a vaccine called NeuroVax, from Immune Response Corporation. Researchers hope the vaccine, which uses protein fragments from T cells, will replenish T reg cells and halt or diminish immune system attacks.

Stem Cell Research

Perhaps the most promise for a "cure" points to stem-cell research. The scientists who called the last century "the century of the gene"—beginning with the discovery of DNA and ending with full mapping of the human genome—now say we are in the "century of the cell and its self-renewal." And that is very promising for people not only with MS, but with Parkinson's disease, rheumatoid arthritis, diabetes, ALS, traumatic spinal cord injury, Purkinje cell degeneration, Duchenne's muscular dystrophy, heart disease, and vision and hearing loss. These, and so many other diseases, we now know, are not the result of a simple microbe or even an individual genetic alteration, but rather the loss of very specific cells.

If you add all the diseases together, we're talking about tens of millions of individuals who have health care needs largely unmet by current medical strategies. This is expected to have a tremendous impact not only on quality of life, but health care costs and overall productivity of our economy. And that's why there's so much incentive to see if the early promise of stem-cell research can be fulfilled.

The hope is that stem cells might be transplanted to target specific cells. In heart disease, stem cells might help grow new heart muscle. In diabetes, stem cells might be transplanted to replace the ones which produce insulin. In the case of MS, the cell that is lost is the oligodendrocyte which helps make myelin. In MS, stem-cell research will try to promote the growth of new myelin, repair damaged cells, or modify the immune system to replace cells that attack myelin. Some research might lead to the development of drugs that could recruit a person's own stem cells to a specific area in the body that needs repair.

There are two types of stems cells used in research:

- *Embryonic stem cells* from leftover embryos created for in vitro fertilization. Fertility doctors create embryos by removing eggs from a woman's fallopian tubes and fertilizing them with sperm in a petri dish. Because of the pain, expense, and high failure rate, doctors usually create more embryos than they can use. Those left over are frozen and, by permission of the donors, can be donated to research. By one estimate, 400,000 embryos are currently stored in clinics across the country. (Less than 3 percent will be donated to research and many will be destroyed.) Embryonic stem cells are very promising because they are *pluripotent*; they can grow into any type of cell in the body. They can also be easily grown in the large numbers needed for stem-cell research and replacement therapies. This is also the case with stem cells taken from umbilical cord blood and placentas.

As long as the embryonic stem cells in a culture are grown under certain conditions, they can remain undifferentiated (unspecialized). If cells are allowed to clump together, forming embryoid bodies, they begin to differentiate spontaneously. They can form muscle cells, nerve cells, perhaps as many as 200 different cell types. Although spontaneous differentiation is a good indication that a culture of embryonic stem cells is healthy, it is not an efficient way to produce specific cell types. The hope is that if scientists can learn how to reliably direct the differentiation of embryonic stem cells into specific cell types, they may be able to use the resulting cells to treat certain diseases.

- *Adult stem cells* are those found in bone marrow and blood. They have also been identified in many organs and tissues, including the brain, skeletal muscle, skin, and liver. In tissue, however, a very small number of stem cells are found. Adult stem cells are generally limited to differentiating into cells of their specific origin. Although not as desirable as the embryonic stem cell, one potential advantage of using adult stem cells is that the patient's own cells could be expanded in a culture and then reintroduced into the patient, eliminating immune system rejection.

The history of research on adult stem cells began about forty years ago. In the 1960s, researchers discovered that bone marrow contains at least two kinds of stem cells. One group, called *hematopoietic stem cells,* forms all the types of blood cells in the body: red blood cells, B lymphocytes, T lymphocytes, natural killer cells, neutrophils, basophils, eosinophils, monocytes, macrophages, and platelets. The second group, called *bone marrow stromal cells*, was discovered a few years later. They can generate bone, cartilage, fat, and fibrous connective tissue.

Also in the 1960s, scientists who were studying rats discovered two regions of the brain that contained dividing cells, which become nerve cells. But it was not until the 1990s that scientists found the adult brain does contain three stem cell types—*astrocytes*, *oligodendrocytes*, and *neurons*, or nerve cells.

In addition, *epithelial* stem cells in the lining of the digestive tract occur in deep crypts and give rise to several cell types: absorptive cells, goblet cells, paneth cells, and enteroendocrine cells. *Skin stem cells* occur in the basal layer of the epidermis and at the base of hair follicles. The epidermal stem cells give rise to keratinocytes, which migrate to the surface of the skin and form a protective layer. The *follicular* stem cells can give rise to both the hair follicle and to the epidermis.

The first scientific experiments with human embryonic stem cells were in 1998 when a group led by Dr. James Thomson at the University of Wisconsin developed a technique to isolate and grow the cells. It took until August 9, 2001 to acquire federal funding. But the funding bill, signed by president George W. Bush, represented a compromise: research would be limited to twenty-two stem-cell lines acquired prior to that date.

The controversy over the public funding of research using human embryos stems from the question of "when does life begin?" Many pro-life advocates believe that a four- to six-day-old embryo in a petri dish is life and should not be destroyed. Others are concerned that growing human embryos will lead to human cloning. Political and ethical debates have been passionate on both sides as embryonic research has continued with private funding only. Public figures such as Michael J. Fox and Nancy Reagan have strongly advocated easing of those stringent laws. Individual states, such as California and Massachusetts, are wrangling their own legislation. And research involving embryonic stem cells is flourishing in other countries with the involvement of some entrepreneurs who are less-than-desirable pioneers.

Currently in the United States, adult stem cells (hematopoietic stem cells, or HSCs) are the only type of stem cell commonly used to treat human diseases. Doctors have been transferring HSCs in bone marrow transplants for over forty years. More advanced techniques of collecting (or "harvesting") HSCs are now routinely used in order to treat leukemia, lymphoma, and several inherited blood disorders. The clinical potential of adult stem cells has also been demonstrated in the treatment of other human diseases that include diabetes and advanced kidney cancer. However, these newer uses have involved studies with a very limited number of patients.

For treatment of MS, early positive signals began with a few leukemia patients who also had MS. Their bone-marrow transplants not only helped their battles with leukemia, their MS symptoms improved as well. By 2005, there were 250 MS patients who underwent bone-marrow transplants. Some online diaries reveal the challenges of bone-marrow transplantation, also called "autologous stem-cell transplantation."

A patient is given infusions of his or her own bone marrow, which has first been extracted and treated. Since no one knows how you get MS or where it might lurk, care is taken to not reinfect the patient with MS. Chemotherapy and sometimes whole-body radiation are also used to wipe out the person's immune system before the treated bone marrow is given back. The treatment requires hospitalization for about a month, during which time the patient can experience fevers, weakness, urinary problems, and infection, until the immune system is built back up. One blogger called Day 17 "hell day." He described a year-long battle to regain his strength and was able to note real stability and improvement in his MS only after about a year.

Most people seeking transplants are those on a rapid, or continuing progressive course, like the blogger. Adult stem-cell transplants have produced some good results, usually for younger, less disabled people. But others have seen their MS return, and with more progression. In some cases patients have died, a sobering reminder that while promising, stem cell research is in its infancy and that the nature of scientific research is responsible trial and error with high risks often preceding the high rewards.

The Cutting Edge

As we go to press, we can also report on the latest reports from the January 2007 international meeting in San Francisco hosted by the National MS Society. There Dr. Anne Baron-Van Evercooren reported that in her Paris laboratory, she and her colleagues have shown that tissues damaged by MS attacks send distress signals which appear to trigger "endogenous" stem cells to start differentiating into immature myelin-making cells. As this is the first step in the body's natural repair process, she sees these stem cells as "candidates of great interest" in research into enhancing myelin repair. "We need to find ways to enhance migration and recruitment by the MS lesions," she told the conference.

Dr. Jeffrey Kocsis and his research team from Yale University have been studying stem cells from the human nose (OECs); cells that produce myelin outside the central nervous system and stem cells found in bone marrow. He reported that surgically transplanted OECs helped in the regrowth of broken axons (nerve fibers) and protected damaged axons. It also helped in remyelination of damaged axons in lab animals. Dr. Kocsis is also working with a group at Tulane University Medical Center on a study of adult stem-cell use to repair spinal cord injury.

Joanne Kurtzburg of Duke University reported on the healing potential of stem cells derived from umbilical-cord blood which can be readily and harmlessly retrieved right after birth. She described success in cord stem-cell transplants in children with neurological disease that may work some day as a strategy for MS.

If you browse online, it's easy to find companies around the world researching, developing, and offering treatment with stem cells. People with MS are seeking stem-cell treatment everywhere from Holland to China, and their testimonials are readily available. One woman interviewed by the BBC said she was able to walk for the first time in thirty-three years. Another company publishes a rating list of observable improvements (from 1 to 20), including many patients who show zero improvement. It is impossible to vet each claim for a treatment that is so new and a disease that is so difficult to predict. And on many of these sites, there is information like this example that can dazzle:

> *Other research has identified, among the many different types of stem cells, one particular type as being especially promising in the treatment of MS. Known as "CD34(+)," these are purified multipotent stem cells known for their ability to migrate to damaged tissue. Related to the CD34(+) stem cell is the "subset" known as the "CD133" stem cell, which has been shown to balance the immune system and*

to differentiate into neuroprotective glia as well as the oligodendrocytes and astrocytes which produce myelin. Such characteristics make the CD34(+) stem cells a particularly potent treatment not only for immune disorders but also in the remyelination of central nervous system diseases. Since MS falls under both categories, these particular stem cells offer great promise for the treatment of MS.

Some information can intrigue . . .

Depression and Stem Cell Therapy:

One of the most common symptoms of Multiple Sclerosis is depression. A new model of depression is now emerging, which is based upon the inhibition of neural stem cell growth within the hippocampal dentate gyrus. Factors such as stress-related glucocorticoids that inhibit stem cell growth also induce depression.

As previously mentioned, it has been shown in animal studies that corticosterone significantly reduces the proliferation of oligodendrocyte precursors throughout the white and gray matter regions of the brain. Since oligodendrocyte precursors play a major role in remyelination, the use of anti-inflammatory therapies may actually perpetuate depression as well as brain injury. In contrast to the use of steroids for treating MS, stem cell therapies promote the proliferation of new oligodendrocytes, with the secondary benefit of alleviating depression. Generally, depression clears within 30 days following CD34(+) stem cell transplantation.

But all must be scrutinized. Let's analyze one more Web page report from the Institute of Cellular Medicine, in Costa Rica, a clinic that offers stem-cell treatments for a variety of diseases. The Web site offers information on its medical staff, along with airline and hotel information and a bit of tourism. One click and you'll find excerpts from reports published in medical journals, all building a case for stem-cell treatment.

> *In a multicenter Phase II study by Fassas and coworkers investigating autologous hematopoietic stem cell transplantation (HSCT) for multiple sclerosis, 85 patients with progressive MS (with a median Extended Disability Status Scale score of 6.5) were treated in 20 European centers. Neurological improvement was seen in 18 patients (21%). Confirmed progression-free survival was seen in 74% of the patients at 3 years. Disease progression was seen in 20%. The authors conclude that autologous HSCT early results are positive and feasible for the management of progressive MS.*

This report is not inaccurate, just incomplete. If, as we did, you look up the original paper by A. Fassas and his team in the November 2002 *Journal of Neurology*, you'll find their experimental high-dose regimen of chemotherapy, growth factors, and stem cells caused seven deaths. Five were from toxicity/infection and two from neurological deterioration. The authors had one more sentence after "early results are positive and feasible." They also concluded, "These multicenter data suggest a significant association with significant mortality risks especially in some patient groups and are being utilized in the planning of future trials to reduce transplant-related mortality." Again, we emphasize that the nature of scientific research is responsible trial-and-error, with high risks often preceding the high rewards. It is not necessary to sanitize the nature of stem-cell research.

A very conservative online site to consult is Quackwatch at www.quackwatch.org. Dr. Stephen Barrett recently published a research project on "the shady side of embryonic stem-cell therapy" in which he reviewed five prominent clinics around the world offering stem-cell therapy, although not the one we addressed in Costa Rica. He concluded, "Although stem-cell therapy has a few practical applications and considerable promise, there is no reason to believe [they] are providing it as a legitimate service. Their theories and methods are simplistic; their treatments may have adverse effects; they offer no credible outcome data; and their promisies go far beyond what is now possible." What's more, he found at least one clinic refused to detail methods for screening against AIDS or hepatitis.

Stem-cell therapy is certainly an exciting and promising direction for people with MS and many other diseases. Still, so much more research is needed to determine if the adult stem-cell mechanisms can, indeed, be identified and controlled, and if existing stem cells from a healthy tissue can be induced to repopulate and repair diseased tissue. Scientists have many basic questions to answer: Does a single type of stem cell exist—possibly in the bone marrow or circulating in the blood—that can generate the cells of any organ or tissue? What are the factors that stimulate stem cells to relocate to sites of injury or damage? Why can embryonic stem cells proliferate for a year or more in the laboratory without differentiating, but most adult stem cells cannot? What are the factors in living organisms that normally regulate stem-cell proliferation and self-renewal?

Global Immunosuppression

If the monoclonal antibody is considered the "Magic Bullet" *global immunosuppression* is the equivalent of dropping the bomb. Some of these therapies, which suppress not just one target but the entire immune system, have stopped the progression of MS for up to a year. Because global immunosuppression has very toxic side effects and can even be fatal if the patient's white cell count is not monitored very closely, its use remains confined to research experiments. It is up to the individual and doctor to evaluate the risk-benefit ratio. The list that follows represents the more popular immunosuppression therapies in trials today. Many of them are administered in combination with other agents such as ACTH or cortisone, but they will be discussed independently here.

Cyclosporine (Sandimmune)

Cyclosporine is an immunosuppressant drug which has been successfully used to prevent rejection in transplant operations. It has also been proved effective in other autoimmune diseases, such as insulin-dependent diabetes. The drug is known to inhibit activity of T cells, so in theory it should be an effective therapy for MS. Preliminary studies showed Cyclosporine to have questionable benefit in MS, but because it is such a valuable immunosuppressant in other situations, a twelve-center study funded by Sandoz Pharmaceuticals, Inc., its manufacturer, is now in progress in the United States and Canada. Although the drug does have a variety of side effects, it does not appear to increase the risk of cancer.

Chlorambucil (Leukeran)

Chlorambucil is another immunosuppressant drug, and may be the best choice because it has less toxicity than the others. It is administered by pulse therapy, a high dose once a month for two days. The patient's white blood cell count must be closely monitored. I have given Chlorambucil to my own patients, who have shown reversal of worsening conditions, as well as slow improvement. While some patients only improved over a short term, others have shown prolonged improvement.

Plasmapheresis

Plasmapheresis is a procedure in which blood is removed from the individual, "cleansed" to remove the lymphocytes, and returned to the body. While the American Academy of Neurology has recently cast doubt on its usefulness in the treatment of MS, there are occasional cases, one of which I have observed personally, that have shown dramatic positive results. This is a tedious and painful procedure to undergo because of the number and duration of the treatments. However, it is a treatment that has worked in desperate situations when all else has failed.

Intravenous Immunoglobulin (IVIg)

Intravenous immunoglobulin is used to treat certain autoimmune diseases that cause peripheral neuropathy. It is sometimes used in desperate cases of MS when rapid worsening is occurring. The drug is given intravenously once a day for three days every two to four weeks. It is very expensive, each infusion costing $2,000.

Newer Treatments

Cladribine (Mylinax)

Cladribine is an immunosuppressant drug used to treat hairy cell leukemia and has shown benefits for people with remitting-relapsing and progressive MS, both primary and secondary. Mylinax appears to stop metabolism in normal and malignant lymphocytes, some known to damage myelin. Although cladribine produced and sustained significant reductions in number and volume of new enhancing lesions, the drug did not improve scores on the disability scales. Still, it has been designated by the FDA as a "fast track" product.

Methotrexate

Methotrexate is a synthetic immunosuppressant used in the treatment of cancer and rheumatoid arthritis, also an autoimmune disease. Early clinical studies showed that methotrexate reduces lesion area in patients with primary-progressive MS but did not produce changes in the disability scale. Although trials in the 1970s did not show promise, there has been a renewed interest after a small study showed a low dose helped deterioration in arm function, although not in leg function.

Alemtuzumab

Alemtuzumab is a monoclonal antibody usually classified as an immunosuppressant. In a study of 29 secondary-progressive MS patients who received a five-day pulse of the drug, alemtuzumab improved MRI and clinical markers of disease for at least eighteen months following treatment. However, 15 patients continued to experience progressive disability. More ominously, one third of treated patients developed autoimmune hyperthyroidism. In early active relapsing-remitting MS, the drug reduced relapses 75 percent and the risk of disability 60 percent, compared to interferon beta-1a. However, 3 patients developed ITP, a condition that reduces platelet count and may cause abnormal bleeding. One patient died.

Use of alemtuzumab has been temporarily suspended, while dosing and toxicity issues are addressed.

Earlier Trials of Chemotherapy Agents

Many chemotherapeutic agents have undergone clinical trials, some have been used in uncontrolled studies, and most remain controversial due to mixed results and severe side effects that include risk of infection, sterility, mutations, hair loss, nausea, and increased risk of cancer. For the most part, a newer drug, Novantrone, is a better choice. But here are other options.

Cyclophosphamide (Cytoxan) is currently being studied for those with rapidly progressing disease. Cyclosporine A, best known as a drug that significantly reduced rejection rates in organ transplants, has been studied and found to slow disease progression, but not enough to change performance of daily activities. Azathioprine (Imuran) is commonly used in rheumatoid arthritis and some cancers. The benefits of these drugs must be weighed against their risks.

Immune System Modifiers

While immunosuppressants diminish the immune system response, other therapies change, or modify, the response. In earlier editions of this book, interferon treatment was listed in this chapter as a "new hope." It is now widely used with great success to alter the course of MS. Here is the next wave of promising therapies.

FTY720

FTY720 (oral fingolimod, from Novartis Pharmaceuticals Corporation) is a promising oral immune system modifier.

A study in relapsing-remitting MS showed more than a 77 percent decrease in annual relapse rates after two years, compared with a placebo. The percentages of relapse-free patients and those without enhancing lesions on MRI were also notable, both greater than 80 percent.

Laquinimod

Laquinimod is another oral immunomodulator under investigation. It is similar in structure to Roquinimex, a compound whose development was halted due to occurrence of serositis and myocardial infarction. Laquinimod inhibited the development of EAE in mice. Patients with MS who participated in a twenty-four-week trial of the drug had a 44 percent reduction in the number of active lesions. In a forty-eight-week study, using a higher dose, 77 percent of patients remained relapse-free during the course of the study.

Rituxan (Rituximab)

Rituxan is a drug that targets B cells, the white blood cells that make antibodies. Researchers began recruiting volunteers with primary-progressive MS in 2006 after earlier, smaller studies showed promise. But since symptoms of primary-progressive MS often appear slowly, it will take a few years before this drug, and others in development for primary-progressive, can be evaluated.

BG000112

BG00012, an oral agent (fumarate from Biogen Idec), was recently studied in a multicenter phase II controlled clinical trial and produced a 69 percent reduction in active inflammation verified by MRIs of 257 people with a relapsing-remitting course.

Oral Teriflunomide

Oral teriflunomide, an agent that modulates T cells, was shown to reduce new lesions seen on MRI by up to 85 percent in a phase II study of 127 patients. A larger study is now underway.

New Treatment for Symptoms

Fampridine-SR (4-AP)

Fampridine-SR is an oral drug designed to give relief of symptoms by compensating for lost nerve conduction. Acorda Therapeutics, in Hawthorne, New York, is expected to seek FDA approval after positive results of a placebo-controlled study of 301 patients with all forms of MS. The company reports an average walking speed increase of 25 percent over the placebo.

This drug is a potassium channel-blocking agent that mimics the effects of cooling and improves nerve conduction, particularly in temperature-sensitive subjects. As 4-AP, it first came on the scene at a 1986 meeting of the American Neurological Association. Back then, two studies showed the drug offered temporary improvements, notably in vision, strength, and coordination. 4-AP is used by an estimated 10,000 people with MS. It has been available by prescription through compound pharmacies, those which offer specially made formulations prescribed by physicians.

Searching for the "MS Virus"

There are three ways an "MS virus" could trigger the immune system response: (1) *a direct virus attack,* (2) *a bystander effect,* or (3) an *immunological cross-reaction.*

There is no evidence that the immune system is triggered by either a direct virus attack or a bystander effect, in which the virus would be so sequestered in the myelin sheath that the immune system would chew at the nervous system to get at the virus, destroying myelin, which happens to be in the way. However, there is some evidence of an immunological cross-reaction between the virus and myelin, which are both made up of chemicals. If the immune system has a poor recognition factor built in, it may not be able to tell the difference between viruses and myelin. So, as soon as the virus sets oft the immune system to chase after it, it chews away at the virus and then goes after the myelin. This is called *molecular mimicry,* and it allows us to believe that certain viruses have biochemical sequences that overlap with myelin proteins and can trigger an autoimmune reaction. There is some preliminary evidence from animal studies that it can work that way. Molecular mimicry may also explain why scientists have failed to uncover the "MS virus." Once cross-reaction to a myelin protein occurs, it is no longer necessary for a virus to be present. The virus is gone, but the immune system, now sensitized to myelin, can repeat the cycle of attacks without it. Still, until there is real documentation that this occurs, scientists will continue to look for an "MS virus," with a focus on the so-called slow viruses.

The Last Mile of the MS Research Marathon

If we are so close, what is it going to take to find the cure for MS? As in all such research, we need three final elements: persistence, a bit of luck, and a brilliant observer.

Most great discoveries have been dependent on the persistence of one researcher who painstakingly reviewed past results and played with all the pieces of the puzzle until they fit together. This is how L-dopa was discovered as a treatment for Parkinson's disease. For at least fifteen years it was well known in Parkinson's research that some brain cells had a deficiency in a neurotransmitter called dopamine. But since all attempts to give dopamine to patients showed no effect, most scientists felt the dopamine deficiency was just a red herring—except for Dr. George Cotzias, a researcher who said to himself, If dopamine doesn't help Parkinson's disease, then all the rules of scientific evidence are worthless. First he tried administering dopamine in the form of dextrodopamine, but it didn't get to the brain. Then he tried it in the form of levodopamine and some got into the brain. Finally, he discovered if he gave levodopamine in high doses, enough could get to the brain to have dramatic results. It was Cotzias's persistence that paid off.

The success of any research also depends on a little old-fashioned serendipity—making discoveries by accident. Ultimately, this serendipity needs a brilliant observer. Think of how Alexander Fleming discovered penicillin. He accidentally spilled mold in his bacteria culture plate and realized something very important occurred that destroyed the bacteria. Accidents just like this probably happened in the labs of many other researchers around the world who probably tossed the culture plate in the trash, thinking it was ruined. It took a brilliant observer like Fleming to know he'd struck gold.

At this point in research, we have money and we have talent. We can always use more of each, but with persistence, good observation, and serendipity, we'll have a cure for multiple sclerosis in the near future. MS research involves many different experts in neurology, virology, immunology, epidemiology, and genetics. There is no one scientist who is an expert in all these fields, and, unfortunately, no one is coordinating all the scientific thought. The questions must be tackled from all their different angles, but eventually someone will have to merge all the information.

Finally, it's important to note that when a cure is found it will help all people with MS. There is good evidence that MS damage can be reversed, that nerve fibers can conduct again if the toxic agent is removed, allowing myelin to regrow, and if nutrients that may have leaked out through the myelin gap are supplied to nerve fibers. With MS research, there is good hope for old and new patients alike.

MS is a job for a master detective. When the final clue is uncovered, six pieces of the mystery puzzle must satisfactorily fit.

1. Myelin damage: What is it that selectively attacks this fatty-protein insulating substance and why?
2. Age of onset: Why does MS almost always begin between the ages of ten and sixty?
3. Geographical distribution: Why does the incidence of MS increase the farther one goes from the equator?
4. Episodic course: What could it be that attacks and goes away?
5. Antibodies in the spinal fluid: Are these a cause or a result of myelin damage?
6. Genetic susceptibility: Why do some people get MS and others don't?

Who is the master detective who will solve the mystery? A basic scientist? A practicing doctor? It might even be a patient. That's not as farfetched as it sounds. One Canadian woman named Sylvia Hall, who was diagnosed as having

MS in 1980, has led scientists down a very intriguing research path. Not only did she and her sister develop MS, she knew of six more girls from their high school who had the disease. Subsequent investigations revealed that, in all, twenty-seven people who lived within five miles of the little Saskatchewan town of Henribourg (population 300) during the 1940s, developed the disease. Today only one person with MS actually lives in Henribourg, so had it not been for the detective work of Sylvia Hall, it is doubtful scientists would have discovered this "hot spot." In the rest of the province, the incidence of MS is 115 per 100,000. In Henribourg the incidence could be calculated at 9,000 per 100,000. In 1983 scientists at the University of Saskatchewan agreed to investigate the conditions of the town before and during World War II, when the Hall sisters and their friends were in high school together (prior to age fifteen). They interviewed people who lived there, took extensive soil and water samples, and are still pursuing the lead. No one knows what might actually be discovered in Henribourg; the point is that one woman with MS, who wrote to universities all over Canada to stir up interest in her discovery, could conceivably make a difference.

We are clearly on the verge of a cure for MS. Whether the immune system response is the cause or the result of the disease, we can now modulate it—tune it up one way or another. In 2006 the National MS Society invested over $42 million in 350 new and ongoing MS research projects. The National Institutes of Health budgets about $110 million a year for MS, and pharmaceutical company studies add even more research dollars.

Hundreds of studies are going on simultaneously across the country and around the world. Researchers from University of California, Los Angeles, reported that Androgel, a testosterone gel, significantly improved cognitive function and slowed brain tissue loss, the conclusion of the first large-scale trial of a sex hormone treatment for MS that followed 130 women with early relapsing-remitting MS. Further studies will involve larger numbers of patients.

Harvard investigators report that people exposed to the Epstein-Barr virus, which causes infectious mononucleosis, were two times as likely to develop MS up to twenty years later.

Stanford University researchers are looking into the role of osteopontin, a protein that is a suspected link to repeated relapses and progression. What's more, the NMSS is bringing researchers together regularly to swap information and move the research as quickly as possible to the patient. November 2006 was the first meeting of fifty members of the four "Nervous System Repair" teams who have a commitment of over $15 million from the NMSS. Here is a roundup from some of their reports:

- Drs. Susumu Mori, Seth Smith, and Daniel Reich reported on new MRI software on stronger MRI magnets to create pictures of fiber tract pathways in MS patients' brains and spinal cords. "These pictures may allow us to better image lesions (damaged areas) and discriminate damage to the axon from damage to myelin, rather than just seeing the inflammation."
- At Johns Hopkins, Drs. Peter Calabresi and Avindra Nath determined that proteins released by immune T cells not only cause damage to nerve cells, but they inhibit nerve precursor cells that are trying to repair the brain. "By understanding which of these proteins is most important we may be able to better dampen the bad inflammation and allow natural reparative processes to occur more efficiently."
- At the University of Wisconsin, Madison, Dr. Ian D.

Duncan's team has isolated oligodendrocytes (myelin-making cells) from stem cells and succeeded in coaxing them to specialize (differentiate) into oligodendrocytes in increasing numbers and percentage using selective growth factors. They have also shown that these cells make myelin when transplanted into animals that are myelin-deficient, thus proving their functional capabilities.

- At Cambridge University in England, Dr. Charles ffrench-Constant's team is working on new therapies to promote repair by remyelination. Dr. Robin Franklin of Cambridge has worked with Dr. David Rowitch of New York's Dana-Farber Cancer Institute to complete a genome scale screen of the myelin repair process, examining over 1,000 transcription factors. They will now focus on twenty-five factors to establish exactly when and where they are expressed during myelin repair.
- Drs. Samuel Weiss (University of Calgary) and Jack Antel (Montreal Neurological Institute) have identified techniques to grow large numbers of human oligodendrocytes, enabling researchers to test drugs directly on human myelinating cells.
- Two classes of nerve-protecting compounds will be tested in two single therapy clinical trials in the United Kingdom. Lamotrigine (currently used to prevent seizures in people with epilepsy) is being tested to see if it can prevent or slow progressive shrinking of the brain (atrophy) in people with secondary-progressive MS. This trial is being run by Dr. Raj Kapoor of the National Hospital for Neurology and Neurosurgery, Queen Square, London.
- The second is a large, multicenter study to see if the active compound in cannabis, THC (tetrahydrocan-

> nabinol) can slow the progressive phase of the disease, as has been suggested in EAE. This is being coordinated at the Peninsula Medical School in Plymouth, England.

Other teams are aggressively looking at epidemiology, genetics, and improvements in existing treatments. Pharmaceutical companies are aggressively trying to improve upon the success of disease-modifying drugs while lessening all side effects down to the irritation at the injection site. Of course, all eyes are still on stem-cell research. It is critical to resolve political and ethical issues.

12

What to Do Until the Cure Comes

It's great that the cure is around the corner, but what are you going to do until the MS mystery is solved? Besides our suggestions of how to stay in top physical and emotional form, there's still a lot more you can do—for yourself and for others. The key is to be resourceful.

Should You Participate in a Research Program?

With so much research under way, many scientists are complaining that all the "virgins" are gone. They are referring to individuals who haven't been exposed to any previous treatment that might affect a new trial. Test subjects are in great demand, and many people with MS are anxious to seek promising new therapies. But the decision to participate in a research program must not be taken lightly. As in any experiment, long-term benefits and side effects are unknown—that's why they have to be tried out on you. No matter how noble your intentions, you must take all aspects of your personal situation into consideration and discuss them in detail with your personal physician, who can help you evaluate the pros and cons. If you'd like to have more children, for example, it's probably best to stay clear of experimental therapies that may cause sterility. Still, not all tests involve therapies with toxic side effects. Some, such as the studies of polyunsaturated fatty acids, just involve taking diet supplements. Others simply test well-known drugs for other symptoms.

If you decide that you would like to participate in a research program, you will need a strong commitment to the scientific process. The tests may be time consuming and may require years of follow-up examinations. Worse, the tests may not only be time consuming but at the end of six months or a year you will learn you only received the placebo. It's also important to understand that you may not be eligible for the next trial that comes down the pike.

Each study is geared toward either relapsing-remitting *or* secondary-progressive MS. Researchers may design a particular trial to include a specific age, sex, DSS disability rating, or even a particular symptom. So don't be disappointed if you're not right for a particular study. Be assured that you're more in demand than you know. But also keep in mind that the study best suited for your situation might not be in your neighborhood. Unless you have your own resources (not to mention motivation) to live close to the medical center where a particular trial is taking place, you're going to have to hold tight. It's more important for research funding to go directly to the investigation than to your living expenses.

Keeping up to date on current research trends is up to you. For many this is an important reason to see their neurologists every six months, even if their personal situations have not changed. This is also a reason to make sure to choose a neurologist who keeps on top of the latest information. There has been an explosion of information in just the last few years, and it's still coming in fast and furious. Make sure your neurologist is in contact with nearby research facilities. Usually, when a study is gearing up, scientists will contact local neurologists in order to enlist patients. If you are interested in participating in a future project, you must let your own doctor know about this so he or she can keep an eye out for a suitable program. If you don't feel your neurologist is supplying you with enough information, consult directly with a neurologist at a research facility.

Go online, but be discerning. Understand, for instance, that Wikepedia, the online encyclopedia, allows ordinary browsers to add information, and not all of it is accurate. There is a difference between that site and the *New England Journal of Medicine*, which publishes professional papers that have undergone a peer review, an evaluation of methodology and analysis by independent experts. We highly recommend the Web site of the National Multiple Sclerosis Society, www.nationalmssociety.org. The NMSS is a solid clearinghouse for information. Its Web site is well designed and easy to navigate. From general information to articles in foreign medical journals to the latest clinical trials to breaking news, it's online. A podcast of the January 16 to 19, 2007 stem-cell research summit was online daily, within hours of the presentations. A few months before, the NMSS site reported on a groundbreaking study from the GAMES group (Genetic Analysis of Multiple Sclerosis in Europeans), a collaborative of some nineteen research groups screening the entire genome, seeking possible markers or genetic sequence variations that show up with higher frequency in patients or family members with a history of MS. Here's a sample of what you'll find online:

> *For this study, the group combined those results and did more in-depth analysis of 17 of the*

most promising markers. Five of the markers turned out to be in the previously known MHC area, and 12 appeared in other areas. These markers were tested against the genetic material of 937 family "trios," 3-person units that include one affected person and both parents. After multiple crosschecking and retesting, the group identified a significant association in the "JAG1" and "POU2AF1" genes.

The JAG1 gene encodes for "jagged 1," a protein that is involved in determining how much repair occurs to myelin, which is a nerve-insulating tissue attacked during MS. POU2AF1 is involved in regulating the activity of immune B cells, which produce antibodies that can contribute to the disease course.

"This is a significant step forward in the search for genes that make people susceptible to developing MS," said Dr. John Richert, Executive Vice President of Research and Clinical Programs at the National MS Society. "What's intriguing is that we know enough now from basic research into the disease to understand how these two candidate genes could indeed play a role, and this encourages more research into their underlying mechanisms," he continued.

The GAMES effort is one of several going on around the world to identify genes related to MS. The National MS Society funds a DNA Bank to further this work, as well as the International MS Genetics Consortium and other research projects. If successful, it would give scientists a roadmap to the cause of MS, as well as to concrete targets for new therapies, the development of diagnostic kits that will help in the early diagnosis of MS, and possibly even ways to prevent the disease.

The National Multiple Sclerosis Society

On May 1, 1945, Sylvia Lawry placed an ad in the *New York Times* to help her brother who had multiple sclerosis. It read, "Multiple sclerosis—will anyone recovered from it please communicate with patient." About fifty people responded, and although none were "recovered," all agreed that an organization was needed to coordinate their efforts. After that response, Sylvia Lawry founded the National Multiple Sclerosis Society. In 1967 she also helped to found the International Federation of Multiple Sclerosis Societies, which today has forty-three member countries actively exchanging ideas. For a complete list of international organizations, member and non-member, log on to www.msif.org or see the listings in the back of this chapter.

Since its founding over sixty years ago, the NMSS has expended over $500 million to advance research. According to its public information, its nationwide income in 2005 was $207 million. Less than 3 percent of that income is from pharmaceutical companies and was received in the form of grants.

Its stated mission is simple: to end the devastating effects of the disease on behalf of the 400,000 Americans who have MS, and their families. To that end, it has a staff of 1,250 paid employees, supplemented by 468,530 positions filled by volunteers who carry out the NMSS daily operations. The Society has 500,000 members including 342,000 individuals who have MS.

The Society partners with the health care community to promote quality health care and serves over one million people annually. A twenty-four-hour services hotline is available by calling 1-800-FIGHT MS. Its website is now counting 54,000 visitors a day.

According to its public information, 78 percent of Society income is devoted to research, while 22 percent goes to support services such as fund raising and management. The Society estimates it costs less than fifteen cents to raise one dollar. In 2005, the Society spent more than $40 million to support over 350 research projects internationally. In addition, it spent more than $114 million to improve the lives of those with MS. "We have been at the core of virtually every major breakthrough in treating and understanding the disease during the last sixty years." The funding of research grants is an intricate process that involves peer review and approval by a committee of scientists and lay board members. In addition to research grants, the society aggressively funds postdoctoral fellowships to interest up-and-coming scientists in the study of MS. "Fifteen years ago we couldn't find scientists who wanted to work on MS. They thought, Why work on MS? There's no Nobel Prize in it. Now it's all changed," said Thor Hanson, president emeritus of the NMSS. Today, because the cure is within our grasp, the society is helping to draw some of the most brilliant young minds to MS research.

Public education is another important goal of the society. Its magazine, *Inside MS,* carries articles on everything from scientific discovery to human interest stories. It is also where individuals can learn about new research programs seeking candidates. We feel it is a very good publication, although some people find that the abundance of ads for wheelchairs and other such aids makes it seem geared toward more advanced forms of MS.

The society also takes an aggressive advocacy role in federal issues relating to people with MS. When the postal rate subsidy for nonprofit organizations was threatened, it lobbied on Capitol Hill to preserve it. After all, just think of the annual mailing costs of valuable information requested by people with MS and their families. In one year alone the society sent out 22 million copies of "What is MS?"—and that's only one of its many popular brochures. And when the Reagan administration tried to cut back National Institutes of Health research funding, lobbyists helped reach a higher compromise figure. The Society's Action Alert Program keeps members informed on pending legislation that affects people with MS. When needed, the society has joined forces with coalitions including the National Health Council, the National Coalition of Immune System Disorders, the Ad Hoc Group for Medical Research Funding, the National Association for Biomedical Research, and the Alliance of NonProfit Mailers.

About two-thirds of the chapters have a professional service person on staff to help with short-term counseling needs. The rest have an area consultant on call. For some people, support groups are a real blessing. They learn to express their feelings and deal with them in an environment of people sharing similar experiences. For others, however, this can produce more anxiety than support. Some groups combine people in remission and without residual symptoms with those who are more disabled. As this can be frustrating to both, many (but not all) chapters are now tailoring the groups to individual needs and offer separate counseling for the newly diagnosed, those who become disabled, couples, and even children. Some chapters are now offering information and education meetings for those not willing to go to a support group. It's a good idea to investigate what your local chapter offers before deciding to join.

On the local level, advocacy is geared toward helping the individual to deal with "the system" and to avoid the red tape of various government agencies such as the Veterans and Social Security Administrations.

While the society helps members in many situations, you should not expect it to solve all your problems. For instance, it cannot pay for medical care or give legal assistance.

For further information, contact:

National Multiple Sclerosis Society
733 Third Avenue
New York, NY 10017
1-800-FIGHT-MS
www.nationalmssociety.org

Appendix 1: Chapters of the National Multiple Sclerosis Society

Alabama Chapter
3840 Ridgeway Drive
Birmingham, AL 35209
Tel: 205-879-8881
Fax: 205-879-8869
E-mail: ALC@NMSS.ORG

Allegheny District Chapter
1040 Fifth Avenue, 2nd Floor
Pittsburgh, PA 15219
Tel: 412-261-6347
Fax: 412-232-1461
E-mail: PAX@NMSS.ORG

Arizona Chapter
315 South 48th Street, Suite 101
Tempe, AZ 85281
Tel: General Public # 480-968-2488
*IRC Bypass # 480-968-2489
Fax: 480-966-4049
E-mail: AZA@NMSS.ORG

Blue Ridge Chapter
One Morton Drive, Suite 106
Charlottesville, VA 22903
Tel: 434-971-8010
Fax: 434-979-4475
E-mail: VAB@NMSS.ORG

Central New England Chapter
101A First Avenue, Suite 6
Waltham, MA 02451
Tel: 781-890-4990
Fax: 781-890-2089
E-mail: MAM@NMSS.ORG

Central North Carolina Chapter
2211 West Meadowview Road, Suite 30
Greensboro, NC 27407
Tel: 336-299-4136
Fax: 336-855-3039
E-mail: NCC@NMSS.ORG

Central Pennsylvania Chapter
2040 Linglestown Road, Suite 104
Harrisburg, PA 17110
Tel: 717-652-2108
Fax: 717-652-2590
E-mail: PAC@NMSS.ORG

Central Virginia Chapter
2112 West Laburnum Avenue, Suite 204
Richmond, VA 23227
Tel: 804-353-5008
Fax: 804-353-5595
E-mail: VAR@NMSS.ORG

Colorado Chapter
700 Broadway, Suite 808
Denver, CO 80203
Tel: 303-831-0700
Fax: 303-831-8001
E-mail: COC@NMSS.ORG

Delaware Chapter
Two Mill Road, Suite 106
Wilmington, DE 19806
Tel: 302-655-5610
Fax: 302-655-0993
E-mail: DED@NMSS.ORG

Eastern North Carolina Chapter
3101 Industrial Drive, Suite 210
Raleigh, NC 27609
Tel: 919-834-0678
Fax: 919-834-9822
E-mail: NCT@NMSS.ORG

Gateway Area Chapter
1867 Lackland Hill Parkway
St. Louis, MO 63146
Tel: 314-781-9020
Fax: 314-781-1440
E-mail: info@Mos.nmss.org

Georgia Chapter
455 Abernathy Road NE, Suite 210
Atlanta, GA 30328
Tel: 404-256-9700
Fax: 404-256-3660
E-mail: GAA@NMSS.ORG

Greater Connecticut Chapter
705 North Mountain Road, Suite G102
Newington, CT 06111
Tel: 860-953-0601
Fax: 860-953-0602
E-mail: CTN@NMSS.ORG

Greater Delaware Valley Chapter
1 Reed Street, Suite 200
Philadelphia, PA 19147
Tel: General Public # 215-271-1500
*IRC Bypass # 215-271-2400
Fax: 215-271-6122
E-mail: PAE@NMSS.ORG

Greater Illinois Chapter
910 West Van Buren Street, 4th Floor
Chicago, IL 60607
Tel: General Public # 312-421-4500
Fax: 312-421-4544
E-mail: ILD@NMSS.ORG

Greater North Jersey Chapter
1 Kalisa Way, Suite 205
Paramus, NJ 07652
Tel: 201-967-5599
Fax: 201-967-7085
E-mail: NJB@NMSS.ORG

Greater Washington Chapter
192 Nickerson Street, Suite 100
Seattle, WA 98109
Tel: General Public # 206-284-4236
*IRC Bypass # 206-284-4254

Fax: 206-284-4972
E-mail: WAS@NMSS.ORG

Hampton Roads Chapter
405 South Parliament Drive, Suite 105
Virginia Beach, VA 23462
Tel: 757-490-9627
Fax: 757-490-1617
E-mail: VAX@NMSS.ORG

Indiana State Chapter
7301 Georgetown Road, Suite 112
Indianapolis, IN 46268
Tel: 317-870-2500
Fax: 317-870-2520
E-mail: INI@NMSS.ORG

Inland Northwest Chapter
818 East Sharp
Spokane, WA 99202
Tel: 509-482-2022
Fax: 509-483-1077
E-mail: WAI@NMSS.ORG

Kentucky/Southeast Indiana Chapter
11700 Commonwealth Drive, Suite 500
Louisville, KY 40299
Tel: General Public # 502-451-0014
*IRC Bypass # 502-267-8487
Fax: 502-451-9747
E-mail: KYW@NMSS.ORG

Lone Star Chapter
8111 North Stadium Drive, Suite 100
Houston, TX 77054
Tel: 713-526-8967
Fax: 713-394-7422
E-mail: TXH@NMSS.ORG

Long Island Chapter
40 Marcus Drive, Suite 100
Melville, NY 11747
Tel: 631-864-8337
Fax: 631-864-8342
E-mail: NYH@NMSS.ORG

Louisiana Chapter
4613 Fairfield Street
Metairie, LA 70006
Tel: General Public # 504-832-4013
*IRC Bypass # 504-210-0932
Fax: 504-831-7188
E-mail: LAM@NMSS.ORG

Maine Chapter
170 US Route One #200
Falmouth, ME 04105
Tel: General Public # 800-FIGHTMS
*IRC Bypass # 207-781-7960
Fax: 207-781-7961
E-mail: MEM@NMSS.ORG

Maryland Chapter
11403 Cronhill Drive, Suite E
Owings Mills, MD 21117
Tel: 443-641-1200

Fax: 443-641-1201
E-mail: MDM@NMSS.ORG

Michigan Chapter
21311 Civic Center Drive
Southfield, MI 48076
Tel: 248-350-0020
Fax: 248-350-0029
E-mail: MIG@NMSS.ORG

Mid-Atlantic Chapter
9801-I Southern Pine Boulevard
Charlotte, NC 28273
Tel: 704-525-2955
Fax: 704-527-0406
E-mail: NCP@NMSS.ORG

Mid America Chapter
P.O. Box 2292
Shawnee Mission, KS 66201
Tel: General Public # 913-432-3926
*IRC Bypass # 913-432-3927
Fax: 913/432-6912
E-mail: KSG@NMSS.ORG

Mid Florida Chapter
2701 Maitland Center Parkway, Suite 100
Orlando, FL 32751
Tel: 407-478-8880
Fax: 407-478-8893
E-mail: FLC@NMSS.ORG

Mid-Jersey Chapter
246 Monmouth Road
Oakhurst, NJ 07755
Tel: 732-660-1005
Fax: 732-660-1338
E-mail: NJM@NMSS.ORG

Mid South Chapter
4219 Hillsboro Road, Suite 306
Nashville, TN 37215
Tel: 615-269-9055
Fax: 615-269-9470
E-mail: TNS@NMSS.ORG

Minnesota Chapter
200 12th Avenue South
Minneapolis, MN 55415
Tel: 612-335-7900
Fax: 612-335-7997
E-mail: MNM@NMSS.ORG

National Capital Chapter
2021 K Street NW, Suite 715
Washington, DC 20006
Tel: 202-296-5363
Fax: 202-296-3425
E-mail: DCW@NMSS.ORG

Nebraska Chapter
Community Health Plaza
7101 Newport Avenue, Suite 304
Omaha, NE 68152
Tel: 402-572-3190

Fax: 402-572-3189
E-mail: NEN@NMSS.ORG

New York City Chapter
733 Third Avenue, 3rd Floor
New York, NY 10017
Tel: 212-463-7787
Fax: 212-986-7981
E-mail: NYN@NMSS.ORG

North Central States Chapter
3800 West Technology Circle, Suite 201
Sioux Falls, SD 57106
Tel: General Public # 605-336-7017
*IRC Bypass # 605-336-6326
Fax: 605-336-8088
E-mail: NDN@NMSS.ORG

North Central Texas Chapter
4086 Sandshell Drive
Fort Worth, TX 76137
Tel: General Public # 817-306-7003
*IRC Bypass # 817-847-6038
Fax: 817-306-7055
E-mail: TXT@NMSS.ORG

North Florida Chapter
4237 Salisbury Road
Bldg. #4, Suite 406
Jacksonville, FL 32216
Tel: 904-332-6810
Fax: 904-332-0898
E-mail: FLN@NMSS.ORG

Northern California Chapter
150 Grand Avenue
Oakland, CA 94612
Tel: General Public # 510-268-0572
*IRC Bypass # 510-267-1934
Fax: 510-268-0575
E-mail: CAN@NMSS.ORG

Northwestern Ohio Chapter
401 Tomahawk Drive
Maumee, OH 43537
Tel: 419-897-9533
Fax: 419-897-9733
E-mail: OHO@NMSS.ORG

Ohio Buckeye Chapter
6155 Rockside Road, Suite 202
Independence, OH 44131
Tel: 800-667-7131
Fax: 216-696-2817
E-mail: OHA@NMSS.ORG

Ohio Valley Chapter
4460 Lake Forest Drive, Suite 236
Cincinnati, OH 45242
Tel: 513-769-4400
Fax: 513-769-6019
E-mail: OHG@NMSS.ORG

Oklahoma Chapter
4606 East 67th Street, Building 7, Suite 103
Tulsa, OK 74136
Tel: 918-488-0882

Fax: 918-488-0913
E-mail: OKE@NMSS.ORG

Oregon Chapter
104 SW Clay Street
Portland, OR 97201
Tel: 503-223-9511
Fax: 503-223-2912
E-mail: ORC@NMSS.ORG

Pacific South Coast
5950 La Place Court, Suite 200
Carlsbad, CA 92008
Tel: 760-448-8400
Fax: 760-804-9266
E-mail: msinfo@mspacific.org

Rhode Island Chapter
205 Hallene Road, #209
Warwick, RI 02886
Tel: 401-738-8383
Fax: 401-738-8469
E-mail: RIR@NMSS.ORG

South Florida Chapter
3201 West Commercial Boulevard, #127
Fort Lauderdale, FL 33309
Tel: 954-731-4224
Fax: 954-739-1398
E-mail: FLS@NMSS.ORG

Southern California Chapter
2440 South Sepulveda Boulevard, Suite 115

Los Angeles, CA 90064
Tel: 310-479-4456
Fax: 310-479-4436
E-mail: CAL@NMSS.ORG

Southern New York Chapter
2 Gannett Drive, Suite LC
White Plains, NY 10604
Tel: 914-694-1655
Fax: 914-694-1656
E-mail: NYV@NMSS.ORG

Upstate New York Chapter
1650 South Avenue, Suite 100
Rochester, NY 14620
Tel: General Public # 585-271-0801
*IRC Bypass # 585-271-0966
Fax: 585-442-2817
E-mail: NYR@NMSS.ORG

Utah State Chapter
6364 South Highland Drive
Salt Lake City, UT 84121
Tel: 801-493-0113
Fax: 801-493-0122
E-mail: UTU@NMSS.ORG

Western Connecticut Chapter
One Selleck Street, Suite 500
Norwalk, CT 06855
Tel: 203-838-1033
Fax: 203-831-2973
E-mail: CTP@NMSS.ORG

Wisconsin Chapter
1120 James Drive, Suite A
Hartland, WI 53029
Tel: 262-369-4400
Fax: 262-369-4410
E-mail: info@wisms.org

Appendix 2: International Federation of Multiple Sclerosis Societies

Associate members and non-member societies are noted.

Argentina
MS Society of Argentina

Name of Society: Esclerosis Múltiple Argentina
Acronym: EMA
Address: Uriarte 1465, (1414) Buenos Aires
Tel: (54) 11 4831 6617
Fax: (54) 11 4831 6786
E-mail: info@ema.org.ar

Armenia
Armenian MS Society

Name of Society: Haykakan crvats sklerozi hasarakutyun
Address: Str. G. Szhdeh 13, Apt. 47, 375006, Yerevan, Republic of Armenia
Tel: (374) 1 44 61 39 or (374) 1 53 03 62
Fax: (374) 1 53 52 96
E-mail: fchilingaryan@yahoo.com
English-Speaking Contact Name: Gayane Muztchyan
English-Speaking Contact E-mail: mgayane@hotmail.com

Australia
National MS Society of Australia

Name of Society: Multiple Sclerosis Australia
Acronym: MSA
Address: c/o Studdy MS Center, Joseph Street, Lidcombe, NSW 2141
Tel: (61) 02 9646 0600
Fax: (61) 02 9646 0675
E-mail: info@mssociety.com.au

Austria
Austrian MS Society

Name of Society: Multiple Sklerose Gesellschaft Österreich
Address: Universitätsklinik für Neurologie, Währinger-Gürtel 18-20, A-1090 Wien
Tel: (43) 1 40 400 3123
Fax: (43) 1 40 400 3141
E-mail: msgoe@gmx.net

Barbados (Non-Member)
MS Society of Barbados

Address: P.O. Box 84, Welches Post Office, St. Michael, Barbados
Tel: (246) 427-1877
E-mail: sandson58@hotmail.com

Belgium
MS Society of Belgium

Name of Society: Ligue Nationale Beige de la Sclérose enPlaques/Nationale Belgische Multiple Sclerose Liga
Address: Rue Auguste Lambiotte 144, bte 8, 1030 Bruxelles
Tel: (32) 2 736 1638

Fax: (32) 2 732 3959
E-mail: ms.sep@ms-sep.be

Belorussia (Non-Member)
Belarisian MS Society

Name of Society: Multiple Sclerosis Association of Belorussia
Acronym: ABRS
Address: Kalinin Strt 7, Belarus 220012, P/c 700802, Minsk
Tel: (375) 17 266 6623
Fax: (375) 17 228 4194
E-mail: russiantarget@solo.by

Bermuda (Non-Member)
The MS Society of Bermuda

Address: Suite 798, 48 Par La Ville, Hamilton, Bermuda HM-09
Tel: 441-293-2649
Fax: 441-232-0699
E-mail: shine@northrock.bm

Bosnia and Herzegovina (Non-Member)
The Association of Societies of People Affected by MS of Bosnia and Herzegovina

Name of Society: Savez udruzenja gradjana oboljelih od multiple skleroze Bosne i Hercegovine
Acronym: SUGOMSBIH
Address: Antuna Branka Simica br. 13, Sarajevo
Tel: (387) 33 65 96 71
Fax: (387) 33 65 96 71
E-mail: msk-sa@bih.net.ba

Brazil

MS Society of Brazil

Name of Society: Associação Brasileira de Esclerose Múltipla
Acronym: ABEM
Address: Avenida Indianópolis, 2752, Indianóplis, São Paulo, SP 04062-003
Tel: (55) 11 5587 6050
Fax: (55) 11 5581 9233
E-mail: diretoria@abem.org.br

Bulgaria (Non-Member)

MS Society Bulgaria Foundation

Acronym: MSSBF
Address: Bulgaria, 1505 Sofia, 17-19, Ivan Milnov str.
Tel: (359) 2 713837
English-Speaking Contact Names: Dessislava Boyadjieva, Alexandra Effisseneva, Christo Balabanov
English-Speaking Contact E-mail: alex@msobshtestvo.org; dessi@msobshtestvo.org

Canada

MS Society of Canada

Name of Society: Multiple Sclerosis Society of Canada / Société canadienne de la sclérose en plaques
Address: 175 Bloor Street East, Suite 700, North Tower, Toronto ON M4W 3R8
Tel: 416-922-6065
Fax: 416-922-7538
E-mail: info@mssociety.ca

Chile (Associate Member)
Chilean Society Against Multiple Sclerosis

Name of Society: Corporación Chilena contra la Esclerosis Múltiple
Acronym: CEM
Address: Diagonal Oriente 1604, Providencia, Santiago
Tel: (56) 2 343 2842
Fax: (56) 2 343 2842
E-mail: jescopelito@emchile.org

Costa Rica (Non-Member)

Name of Society: Asociación Lucha contra la Esclerosis Múltiple de Costa Rica
Acronym: ALCEM
Address: P.O. Box 2028-4050, Alajuela, Costa Rica
Tel: (506) 430 1314
Fax: (506) 296 7613
E-mail: yramirez15@hotmail.com
English-Speaking Contact Name: Yamileth Ramirez

Croatia (Non-Member)
Association of Multiple Sclerosis Societies of Croatia

Name of Society: Savez društava multiple skleroze Hrvatske
Acronym: SDMSH
Address: Trnsko 34, 10000 Zagreb, Croatia
Tel: (385) 1 6554 757
Fax: (385) 1 6552 265
E-mail: sdms_hrvatske@sdmsh.orq

Cuba (Non-Member)
Multiple Sclerosis Cuba

Name of Society: Esclerosis Múltiple Cuba
Acronym: EMCuba

Address: Calle 223 N° 23604, Fontanar, La Habana 19250
Tel: (53) 745 1526
E-mail: emcuba@jagua.cfg.sld.cu
English-speaking contact: Natasha Vázquez
English-speaking contact E-mail: nataliav@enet.cu

Cyprus (Associate Member)
Cyprus Multiple Sclerosis Association
Name of Society: Cyprus Multiple Sclerosis Association
Address: 67-69 Ayiou Nicolaou Street, 2408 Engomi, Nicosia
Tel: (357) 22 590949
Fax: (357) 22 590979
E-mail: multips@logos.net.cy

Czech Republic
Czech Multiple Sclerosis Society
Name of Society: Unie Roska çeská MS spoleçnost
Acronym: CzMSS
Address: P.O. Box 38, 120 00 Praha 2
Tel: (420) 2 4172 8619
Fax: (420) 2 6671 2511
E-mail: alex@msobshtestvo.org

Denmark
Danish Multiple Sclerosis Society
Name of Society: Scelroseforeningen
Address: Mosedalvej 15, DK-2500 Valby
Tel: (45) 36 46 36 46
Fax: (45) 36 46 36 77
E-mail: info@scleroseforeningen.dk

Ecuador (Non-Member)

Name of Society: Fundación Ecuatoriana de EM
Address: Eloy Alfaro #2045 & Suiza, Quito
Tel: (593) 2 444 600
Fax: (593) 2 465 433
E-mail: danibect@impsat.net.ec

Estonia (Non-Member)
Eesti Sclerosis Multiplexi Uhing

Address:Lao 2a-16, Tartu, Estonia 51010
Tel: (372) 507 9153
Fax: (372) 7 318534
E-mail: katring@emh.ee

Finland
Finnish MS Society

Name or Society: Suomen MS-Liitto ry
Address: PL 15 Seppäläntie 90, 21251 Masku
Tel: (358) 2 4392111
Fax: (358) 2 4392133
E-mail: ms-liitto@ms-liitto.fi

France
French MS Society

Name of Society: Ligue Française centre la Sclérose En Plaques
Acronym: LFSEP
Address: 40 rue Duranton, 75015 Paris
Tel: (33) 1 53 98 98 80
Fax: (33) 1 53 98 98 88
E-mail: info@lfsep.asso.fr

Germany
German MS Society

Name of Society: Deutsche Multiple Sklerose Gesellschaft Bundesverband e.V.
Acronym: DMSG
Address: Küsterstrasse 8, 30519 Hannover
Tel: (49) 511 9 68 34 0
Fax: (49) 511 9 68 34 50
E-mail: dmsg@dmsg.de

Greece
Greek Multiple Sclerosis Society

Name of Society: Greek Multiple Sclerosis Society
Address: 2-4 Faethonos Str Thessaloniki 54351
Tel: (30) 23109 49909
Fax: (30) 23109 49909
E-mail: mssoc@hol.gr

Guatemala (Non-Member)
MS Society of Guatemala

Name of Society: Asociación Guatemalteca de Esclerosis Múltiple
Acronym: ASOGEM
Address: 2a. Calle "A" 34-25 Zona 11, Utatlán II, Guatemala City, Guatemala
E-mail: asogem@c.net.gt

Honduras (Non-Member)
Honduran MS Association

E-mail: marcotmedina@yahoo.com
President: Prof. Marco T. Medina

Hungary
Hungarian Multiple Sclerosis Society
Name of Society: Magyar SM Társaság
Address: 8000 Székesfehérvár, Jancsár u.9
Tel: (36) 22 328 454
Fax: (36) 22 328 454
E-mail: smkozpont@albatct.hu

Iceland
MS Society of Iceland
Name of Society: MS Félag Íslands
Address: Sléttluvegur 5, 103 Reykjavik
Tel: (354) 568 8620
Fax: (354) 568 8688
E-mail: msfelag@msfelag.is

India
Multiple Sclerosis Society of India
Name of Society: Multiple Sclerosis Society of India
Acronym: MSSI
Address: No 4 Ground Floor, Shree Laxmi Sadan, 49/50 Gokhale Road (North), Dadar (West) Mumbai—400 028
Tel: (91) 22 437 6855
Fax: (91) 22 444 2067
E-mail: mssindia1@vsnl.com

Iran (Associate Member)
Iranian MS Society
Name of Society: Iranian MS Society
Acronym: IMSS
Address: 58, Vessal-Shirazi Avenue, Vessal, Tehran 1417863811

Tel: (98) 21 6951187
Fax: (98) 21 6499514
E-mail: info@iranms.org

Iraq (Non-Member)
Iraqi Multiple Sclerosis Society
E-mail: luaayabd@yahoo.co.uk
Chief Executive: Luaay A. Waheed

Ireland
MS Society of Ireland
Name of Society: MS Society of Ireland Ltd
Acronym: MSI
Address: MS Resource Centre, 80 Northumberland Road, Dublin 4
Tel: (353) 1 678 1600
(MS Helpline 1850 233 233)
Fax: (353) 1 678 1601
E-mail: info@ms-society.ie

Israel (Associate Member)
Israel MS Society
Name of Society: Israel MS Society
Address: 75 Yehuda Halevi Street, Tel Aviv 65796
Tel: (972) 3 560 9222
Fax: (972) 3 560 9224
E-mail: agudaims@netvision.net.il

Italy
Italian MS Association
Name of Society: Associazione Italiana Sclerosi Multipla
Acronym: AISM
Address: Via Operai 40, 16149 Genoa

Tel: (39) 010 271 3226
Fax: (39) 010 271 3205
E-mail: aism@aism.it

Japan
Japan Multiple Sclerosis Society
Acronym: JMSS
Address: 4-1-2 Kotobuki, Taito-Ku, Tokyo
Tel: (81) 3 3847 3561
Fax: (81) 3 3842 0289
E-mail: jmss@tk.sanyeicorp.co.jp

Jordan (Non-Member)
Address: P.O. Box 950831, 1119 Amman, Jordan

Kazakhstan (Non-Member)
E-mail: adilnmbs@yahoo.com
President: Adil Nurguzhaev

Kuwait (Non-Member)
Acronym: KMSRO
Address: Hali United Group (HUG), P.O. Box 34812, Audillya, 73103 Kuwait
Tel: (965) 900 3336
Fax: (965) 532 2189
E-mail: bashayer@qualitynet.net

Latvia
Latvian MS Association
Name of Society: Latvijas Multiplăs Sklerozes Asociăcija
Acronym: LMSA
Address: Melidas Str 10, Riga, LV-1015
Tel: (371) 7 351 792

Fax: (371) 7 351 792
E-mail: lmsa@lmsa.lv

Lebanon (Non-Member)

Name of Society: Amis Libanais des Scléroses en Plaques
Address: P.O. Box 170, Zahle, Lebanon
E-mail: alsep2000@hotmail.com

Lithuania (Non-Member)
Lithuanian Multiple Sclerosis Union

Address: Erfurto 6-11, Vilnius, 2043, Lithuania
Tel: (370) 2 706 143
Fax: (370) 2 64 29 34
E-mail: info@liss.lt

Luxembourg
MS Society of Luxembourg

Name of Society: Ligue Luxembourgeoise de la Sclérose en Plaques
Acronym: LLSP
Address: An der Bongeschgewan, 48 rue du Verger, L-2665
Tel: (352) 40 08 44
Fax: (352) 40 28 04
E-mail: mslux@pt.lu

Malta (Associate Member)
Multiple Sclerosis Society of Malta

Name of Society: Multiple Sclerosis Society of Malta
Acronym: MSSM
Address: PO Box 209, CMR Valletta
Tel: (356) 21 416 206
Fax: (356) 21 230 538
E-mail: lagius@onvol.net

Mexico (Associate Member)
Mexico MS Society
Name of Society: Esclerosis Múltiple México
Acronym: EMMEX
Address: Av. Fernando No. 68 col Álamos, C.P. 03400, Delegación Benito Juárez, México D.F.
Tel: (52) 33 31 88 26 98
Fax: (52) 33 36 17 75 87
E-mail: emmex-org@hotmail.com

Netherlands
MS Society of the Netherlands
Name of Society: Stichting MS Research
Address: Krimkade 20b, Postbus 200, 2250 AE Voorschoten
Tel: (31) 71 5 600 500
Fax: (31) 71 5 600 501
E-mail: info@msresearch.nl

New Zealand
MS Society of New Zealand
Name of Society: MS Society of New Zealand Inc
Acronym: MSNZ
Address: PO Box 2627, Wellington
Tel: (64) 4 499 4677
Fax: (64) 4 499 4675
E-mail: info@msnz.org.nz

Norway
MS Society of Norway
Name of Society: Multipel Sklerose Forbundet I Norge
Address: Tollbugata 35, N-0157, Oslo
Tel: (47) 22 47 79 90

Fax: (47) 22 47 79 91
E-mail: epost@ms.no

Pakistan (Non-Member)
Multiple Sclerosis Society of Pakistan
Address: 72/A Sindhi Muslim Housing Society, Karachi 74400
Tel: (92) 21 455 2501

Panama (Non-Member)
Juan Rodolfo Santini Foundation/Fundación Esclerosis Múltiple Panamá
Name of Society: Fundación Juan Rodolfo Santini
Acronym: FEMPA
Address: PO Box 0832-1598 WTC, Panama
Tel: 507-265-5237
Fax: 507-265-5237
E-mail: fem_panama@hotmail.com

Paraguay (Non-Member)
E-mail: victhamu@highway.com.py
President: Fernando Hamuy Diaz de Bedoya

Peru (Non-Member)
Association "Multiple Sclerosis Peru"
Name of Society: Asociación "Esclerosis Múltiple Perú"
Acronym: ESMUP
Address: Alameda del Rocío 581 Surco, Lima 33 Perú
Tel: (51) 1 2712876
Fax: (51) 1 2472291
E-mail: postin@terra.com.pe

The Philippines (Non-Member)
MS Society of The Philippines
Address: 20 Purdue Street, Northeast Greenhills, San Juan Metro Manila 1502
E-mail: bsystems@pworld.net.ph

Poland
Polish MS Society
Name of Society: Polskie Towarzystwo Stwardnienia Rozsianego
Acronym: PTSR
Address: ul. Bagatela 13 lok. 43, 00-585 Warszawa, Polska
Tel: (48) 22 856 76 66
Fax: (48) 22 849 10 65
E-mail: biuro@ptsr.org.pl

Portugal
MS Society of Portugal
Name of Society: Sociedade Portuguesa de Esclerose Múltipla
Acronym: SPEM
Address: Rua Zofimo Pedroso, 66, 1950-291, Lisboa
Tel: (351) 21 865 04 80
Fax: (351) 21 865 04 89
E-mail: spem@spem.org

Romania (Associate Member)
National Union of Multiple Sclerosis Foundations of Romania
Name of Society: Uniunea Nationala a Organizatiilor de Multiple Scleroza din Románia
Acronym: UNOMS
Address: 2/B Str Buzaului, CPU OP7 Oradea 3700 Romania

Tel: (40) 259 41 71 36
Fax: (40) 259 40 66 62
E-mail: ssmr@smromania.ro

Russia (Non-Member)
All Russian MS Organization
Acronym: (PRO PwMS)
Address: President Council: Russia, 127273, Moscow, Berezovaja Alley, 7, Room 292
Directorate: Russia, 443090, Samara, Antonova-Ovseenko Street, 53A, Office 200
Tel: (7) 095 4022968, (7) 9272 014705, (7) 8462 246956
Fax: (7) 8462 246956
E-mail: sams03@mail.ru

Saudi Arabia (Non-Member)
Address: Department of Neurosciences—MBC 76, King Faisal Specialist Hospital & Research Centre, P.O. Box 3354, Riyadh 11211
Tel: (966) 1 464 7272 ext 32819
Fax: (966) 1 442 4763
E-mail: boholega@kfshrc.edu.sa

Serbia (Non-Member)
MS Society of Serbia
Name of Society: Drustvo Multiple Skleroze Srbije
Acronym: DMSS
Address: 11000 Belgrade, dr Subotica 6
Tel: (381) 11 361 05 20
Fax: (381) 11 361 05 20
E-mail: Tanya Dakic (contact): tanjadms@eunet.yu

Slovakia
Slovak Multiple Sclerosis Society
Name of Society: Slovenský Zväz Sclerosis Multiplex
Acronym: SZSM
Address: u lenova 12, 917 00 Trnava
Tel: (421) 33 551 3009
Fax: (421) 33 534 4581
E-mail: szsm@stonline.sk

Slovenia
MS Society of Slovenia
Name of Society: Zdruzenje Multiple Skleroze Slovenije
Acronym: ZMSS
Address: Maroltova 14, 1000 Ljubljana
Tel: (386) 1 568 7299
Fax: (386) 1 568 72 97
E-mail: info@zdruzenje-ms.si

South Africa (Non-Member)
Multiple Sclerosis South Africa
Name of Society: Multiple Sclerosis South Africa
Acronym: MSSA
Address: PO Box 91077, Auckland Park, Johannesburg 2006
Tel: (27) 11 482 3280 (Inland branch office)
Fax: (27) 11 482 3283 (Inland branch office)
E-mail: inlchair@jnb.stormnet.co.za

South Korea
Korean Multiple Sclerosis Society
Name of Society: Korean Multiple Sclerosis Society
Acronym: KMSS
Address: 421 Koryo Academitel, 437-3 Ahyoun-dong, Mapo-gu, Seoul, South Korea 121-011

Tel: (82) 2 362 7774
Fax: (82) 2 362 7744
E-mail: kmss@kmss.or.kr

Spain
MS Society of Spain
Name of Society: Asociación Española de Esclerosis Múltiple
Acronym: AEDEM
Address: c/Modesto Lafuente, 8 1st Centro Derecha, 28010, Madrid
Tel: (34) 91 448 1261
Fax: (34) 91 448 1261
E-mail: aedem@aedem.org

Sweden
Swedish Association of Neurologically Disabled
Name of Society: Neurologiskt Handikappades Riksforbund
Acronym: NHR
Address: Box 49084, S-100 28 Stockholm
Tel: (46) 8 677 7010
Fax: (46) 8 241 315
E-mail: nhr@nhr.se

Switzerland
Swiss Multiple Sclerosis Society
Name of Society: Schweizerische Multiple Sklerose Gesellschaft
Address: Josefstrasse 129, Postfach, CH-8031 Zürich
Tel: (41) 43 444 43 43
Fax: (41) 43 444 43 44
E-mail: info@multiplesklerose.ch

Taiwan (Non-Member)
Multiple Sclerosis Association of Taiwan

Acronym: MSTW
Address: No. 10-2, Lane 290, Chung-Nan Rd., Douliou City, Yunlin County, Taiwan, Republic of China
Tel: (886) 5 551 9330
Fax: (886) 5 551 1013
E-mail: ms@ms.org.tw

Turkey
Turkey MS Society

Name of Society: Türkiye Multipl Skleroz Dernegi
Address: Buyukdere Caddesi, Hukukcular Sitesi No 24/21, Mecidiyekoy, Istanbul
Tel: (90) 212 275 2296
Fax: (90) 212 265 9420
E-mail: aunlusoy@superonline.com

Ukraine (Non-Member)
Kharkov Regional Multiple Sclerosis Association

Acronym: KhRMSA
Address: 71 Pobeda Ave., Apt.198, Kharkov 61174
Tel: (380) 057 337 66 80
E-mail: khrmsa@kharkov.ua

United Kingdom
MS Society of Great Britain and Northern Ireland

Name of Society: MS Society of Great Britain and Northern Ireland
Address: MS National Centre, 372 Edgeware Road, London, NW2 6ND
Tel: (44) 020 8438 0700
Fax: (44) 020 8438 0701
E-mail: info@mssociety.org.uk

Uruguay (Associate Member)
Multiple Sclerosis Uruguay

Name of Society: Esclerosis Múltiple Uruguay
Acronym: EMUR
Address: SEDIN, Instituto de Neurología, 2° piso, Hospital de Clínicas, Avenida Italia s/n, Montevideo
Tel: (598) 2 487 1515 ext. 2558
Fax: (598) 2 600 4301
E-mail: emur@adinet.com.uy

Venezuela (Non-Member)

Name of Society: Asociación Venezolana de Esclerosis Múltiple
Address: Apartado 66752, Plaza Las Americas, Caracas 1061–A
E-mail: avem86@cantv.net

Zimbabwe
Multiple Sclerosis Society of Zimbabwe

Name of Society: Multiple Sclerosis Society of Zimbabwe
Acronym: MSSZ
Address: PO Box BE 1234, Beldevere, Harare
Tel: (263) 4 740 472
Fax: (263) 4 740 472
E-mail: therobs@zol.co.zw

Appendix 3: Your Contributions to Research

While some people are fortunate enough to be able to afford generous financial contributions to the National Multiple Sclerosis Society, others are not. If you're among those who can't open their checkbooks as often as they'd like, do not feel frustrated. You can contribute to science in other important ways. First, be politically involved. If you're on the list to receive an Action Alert from NMSS, respond to it. Write to your senators and congressmen when you learn of legislation that will affect people with MS. And act *immediately*. There's no point in your vote being counted after the fact.

Challenge those who protest the use of animals in scientific research. In recent years, fanatical groups have created a ground-swell of sympathy on behalf of animals studied in laboratories. Some groups raid clinics and release animals, ruining years of experiments. Others have chained themselves to clinic gates, threatened scientists, and spread misinformation. Such groups cannot and should not be allowed to interfere with vital research. If *they* contact the local newspapers and write letters to the editor, do the same. If *they* carry protest signs, you should too. Maybe if we carried our own banners, "Would you like to give your child's polio vaccine back?" or "We love animals, but we love our relatives more," the message would come across loud and clear. Animal research should be done under humane conditions, but it *must* be done.

Finally, there is one ultimate contribution that people with MS can and should make—the donation of brain and spinal cord tissue to science after death. One brain can provide enough material for more than one hundred studies. Remember that scientists now have to rely on the animal model, EAE, in research. The study of MS in the human brain is essential in the search for a cure. In Parkinson's disease, studies made possible by brain donors were how the breakthrough in treatment came about.

Anyone eighteen years of age or older may become a donor simply by signing an organ donation card. If you are under eighteen, a parental signature is required. The next of kin may authorize a donation after the person's death, except in the situation where the deceased specified at some time that he or she did not wish to be a donor.

Brain donations do not affect funeral and burial ceremonies in any way; no scars are visible. For the donation to be of maximum value, the brain should be removed within twelve to twenty-four hours of death. The research centers make all the arrangements and cover all expenses. It is best to arrange for the donation as early as possible. You can always change your mind, rip up your donor card, and tell your family of your new decision.

Thousands of people with MS have already signed up to be donors. Normal brains are also much in demand. If you wish to participate, contact any of the three major neurological research centers specializing in the study of MS:

MS Human Neurospecimen Bank
Veterans' Administration Medical Center
11301 Wilshire Boulevard
Los Angeles, CA 90073
Tel: 310-268-3536
Tel: 310-478-3711 after hours
Web site: www.loni.ucla.edu/nnrsb/NNRSB

Rocky Mountain MS Center
Research Divison
701 East Hampden Avenue, Suite 420
Englewood, CO 80110
Tel: 303-788-4030

A Note from the Authors

After Shirley Temple Black invited news camera crews into her hospital room to enlighten others about mastectomy, the perception of breast cancer was never the same. When Betty Ford brought the struggle of her pill and alcohol addiction to the public, the consciousness of a whole nation was raised. Ronald Reagan's colon cancer, Magic Johnson's AIDS, Michael J. Fox's battle with Parkinson's disease—we've learned so much from each celebrity disclosure. Of course, some famous people have MS: actress Teri Garr, Fox News's Neil Cavuto, talk show host Montel Williams, author Joan Didion . . . all active and productive people in the public eye. Legendary comedian Richard Pryor recently died of complications of a more debilitating form of MS and unrelated health problems. But there's never been the one big dramatic media event to bring MS to the public's attention.

This means that the real crusade is up to you. You must be your own role model, have your own courage, and develop your own personal strength. You *can* cope with MS; you haven't yet been given the option not to. We say "yet" because the cure is near. And we look forward with great confidence to the day this book is obsolete—when hearing about MS will be like hearing about "consumption." Until then, *do not* let MS beat you. Process the information you've learned, apply it to the best of your ability, and then tuck this book away in a drawer. The personal triumphs will be yours and yours alone, and they can be incredible.

Index